GET WELL

EVEN WHEN
YOU'VE BEEN TOLD

YOU CAN'T

GET WELL

EVEN WHEN
YOU'VE BEEN TOLD

YOU CAN'T

SIMPLE STEPS FOR FINDING
PERFECT HEALING
USING METHODS OUTSIDE OF
CONVENTIONAL MEDICINE.

SANDY COWEN

Published by Empower Press, Scottsdale, Arizona

Library of Congress Control Number: 2008933547

ISBN: 978-0-9818948-0-5

Printed in the United States of America

Original cover design by Scott Anderson – Phoenix, Arizona.

PUBLISHER'S NOTE

DISCLAIMER

The information presented in this book is provided on an "as is" basis and it is not intended to diagnose, treat, cure or prevent any specific physical or mental condition or disease. It is also not intended as a substitute for the advice and treatment of a licensed medical professional. Its contents reflect the author's own experiences with holistic healing and any views and opinions expressed therein are provided for informational and educational purposes only.

The author is not a licensed medical professional. Consult with your personal healthcare specialist regarding your own medical care. Except as specifically stated, and to the limits allowed by law, the author, publisher and any other contributor to this book disclaim any liability and damages arising, directly or indirectly, from the inappropriate use of the information contained within this book.

This book is dedicated to every individual
who is willing to fight for good health
and a better quality of life.

Contents

Introduction

I was not always an advocate for alternative medicine, a believer in the holistic approach to healing, or stridently committed to conventional medicine in moderation. I didn't grow up with parents who fed me tofu, who disallowed sugar in the home and who routinely wore Birkenstocks. I am the stereotypical self-made business woman who has earned respect from her peers and always enjoyed enormous credibility in the community. I'm very professional, have served on a number of hospital/healthcare boards and don't look like a typical advocate of a message about breaking free from the conventional - but today I am.

This was the beginning. I was adopted at birth and raised in the Midwest by simple, eighth-grade educated parents who were blue-collar, meat and potatoes people. I was not considered a robust child - maybe even a little fragile, health-wise. I was tall and skinny, and I seem to remember I had lots of colds and sniffles. I had the normal battery of childhood diseases: measles, chickenpox, mumps, and of course, the standard tonsillectomy at age six.

As a working adult, I became entrenched in the media and advertising world, which back in the 60's and 70's consisted of two martini lunches, cigarette smoking and a pressure-cooker work life driven by deadlines. By the mid 70's, I had been through a divorce and my lifestyle, at work and at home, was full of stress and bad habits. It was extremely difficult being an undercapitalized small business owner and single mother. A few years later, it was equally tough being a wife, a mother and an overachiever who worked 70-80 hour weeks and didn't take a full-week's vacation for eight years. My lifestyle was a mess that included a poor diet, too little sleep and a family dynamic influenced by a new husband and that resulting challenging relationship.

While I was building my business, struggling with my marriage and trying to be a good mother, I also served on the board of directors for a number of non-profits and for-profits, which included a significant chain of hospitals in Arizona. For that reason, I knew the best doctors in the community and many were my friends. When I needed help I ran to one of them for a quick fix so I could keep pushing my body to do the max. I wasn't raised or conditioned to challenge what my doctors told me and besides I was too busy to do anything but take the prescription and keep running full speed ahead.

By the 1980's my body returned all these favors and began a twenty-year process of delivering difficult conditions which were off-shoots of a lifestyle that weakened my immune system to such an extent that every genetic predisposition I was prone to eventually surfaced. Initially, I did what I was conditioned to do: run to the best medical doctors for a "cure". After a couple of years of trusting in a system that previously accommodated my needs, I finally found myself sick of being sick. I began to lose confidence in the results my doctors provided and I started to look elsewhere.

How did I know what to do, where to go, who to call and which methods to try? I didn't. I relied on faith, and some sort of knowing within me that told me since God had created such an incredible, comprehensive Universe - surely he had created answers somewhere, for everything. Maybe they weren't well known - maybe not medically sanctioned, and maybe not easily accessible - but I knew answers must exist because it seemed *some* people were getting well from these same conditions. My faith was the catalyst. God, or the Universe if you wish, delivered; results followed.

Examples From My Journeys.

Rheumatoid Arthritis

One night in 1981 I awoke about 3:00 AM with excruciating pain in my right knee. I was immobilized for hours, unable to twist my leg or move the muscle that regulated the knee. I thought my cartilage had dislodged. The next day after the pain released, my chiropractor checked my knee for something out of place, but everything seemed fine. Weeks later a similar attack hit my left hip – also in the middle of the night. I had to be carried into my doctor's office because putting weight on that hip generated unbearable pain. I was referred to a rheumatologist; the diagnosis was palendromic rheumatism.

I was told that this condition might eventually transition into rheumatoid arthritis. The physician was right. Some months later, after a rash of similar attacks that eventually became more frequent and longer in duration, I was back in his office, a victim of rheumatoid arthritis (RA). Like others with RA, the expected degenerative, debilitating symptoms plagued me, but in my case they seemed to have come on all too quickly and with a complete vengeance. I was told this disease was incurable but my doctor hoped to minimize the symptoms with medication.

After nearly two years of conventional medical treatment, including daily doses of powerful anti-inflammatory drugs and trips to the emergency room for steroid injections, my physician decided to prescribe a form of chemotherapy, Methotrexate, to quiet my T-cells and thereby mitigate the increasingly painful symptoms. It became apparent to me that I was not really improving - my medications were just getting stronger. Energy-wise, I could only function at work a few hours a day before I returned home, collapsed on the sofa for the rest of the evening and had to be helped into the bathroom or bedroom by my teenage son or my husband. Deformity started in my hands and the swelling, stiffness and pain were unrelenting in nearly every joint in my body. I lost nearly 20 percent of my hair and my skin looked like a woman in her seventies (I was 37 at the time). My body was aging so rapidly I could hardly believe it. This, I thought, was not the way I wanted to live.

At this point I discontinued conventional medicine and took matters into my own hands. I had no idea where I was going to find help but I knew answers must exist somewhere. I was off all medications within months, and began a healing journey that led to marked improvement within the first 90-days. Using nutritional therapy, controlling my systemic candidiasis, adding a number of supplements, making significant lifestyle and attitude changes and getting more rest - within a few years, my immune system was strong enough to fight the disease and win. No drugs, no doctors, no disfigurement and no symptoms. Today I am as flexible and graceful as a dancer, have the skin of a woman many years younger and have healthy looking hair.

Psoriasis

One day my legs began to itch. I thought it was dry skin – but I could feel hardening under the surface and lotions didn't help. The more I scratched the more my skin became irritated. Soon I noticed dry, red scaly patches appearing and when I scratched them, they bled. The diagnosis was psoriasis. It was ugly and terribly difficult to deal with because the itching never seemed to stop. The condition ran from just under my knees to my ankles on both legs. My legs looked horrific and for more than two years I could only wear pants. I was given topical creams but the more I read about the condition and the prognosis, the more discouraged I became. The doctors didn't seem to have a cure, but there was a national association that I could join with others suffering the same condition.

Again, I became discouraged with the answers I got from my doctors. I applied the cream and hoped for the best. "If this doesn't work", they said, "we'll try a different cream". It seemed to me the itching was a symptom of something much deeper, but because the doctors were unconcerned about digging further, I again walked away from traditional treatments.

Once I discontinued all the prescription drugs I had been taking, many of which sped up my metabolism and filled my body with toxins my skin was trying to release, and the psoriasis began to subside. As my immune system became healthier the condition totally disappeared. Emotional work also helped. I have been psoriasis-free for more than twenty-years and my legs now are back to normal.

Chronic Respiratory Issues and Allergies

For nearly ten years, starting from the time I was in my mid-twenties, I was literally plagued by chronic allergies and upper respiratory issues. Colds and more colds, which generally settled in my chest, often resulted in bronchitis, pneumonia or severe colds that drug on for what seemed like forever. I ran to the pulmonary specialist routinely and took daily doses of antihistamines and bronchial drugs, as well as antibiotics at least every month. When my colds or flu symptoms got too bad, I was given steroids to make it possible for me to keep working. As a single mom with a new business, I couldn't afford to be sick.

When the rheumatoid arthritis hit few years later, I was still battling the respiratory symptoms. Then as I began the holistic healing journey, eliminated all my prescription medicines and began the process of making my immune system stronger, everything improved. By the time my arthritis was gone, so were my chronic allergies.

Today, the chronic respiratory issues are history. Once or twice a year I'll begin to catch a cold (with grandkids – that's a given) but my preventive therapies generally stop the process before it progresses into any full-blown condition. Even if I come down with a cold, it is relatively mild and my chest and lungs are not affected. I am so much healthier overall. It is simply amazing!

Leukemia

Tired - I was so tired. But, I figured since I just finished co-chairing a political fundraiser for a presidential candidate in Metro Phoenix and also had a busy work schedule the past few months, I just chalked it up to overwork and over commitment in general.

Over the next several weeks, I grew weaker and neither rest nor sleep seemed to help me rebound. My energy level was in the basement so three months later I decided to go to my holistic physician for a routine physical. That was in late August, 1999.

I received a phone call at home from my doctor telling me my white count looked a little high and she'd like to have me come back for more blood work. I complied and a couple days later she called again to tell me she was very concerned and recommended I see a hematologist. I asked her, "Why - what do you think is the matter?"

"You may have lymphoma or leukemia. You really need to see a specialist," my doctor stated.

I am a tough cookie; I handle stress well and am usually the strong one in the face of crisis but I must tell you this brought me to my knees. I was in shock. I had spent years getting over the rheumatoid arthritis, psoriasis and chronic allergies. I just couldn't understand why this was happening to me now. For the next several hours I walked around the house in a fog and when I intermittently gained enough clarity I'd pick up a book and read about the various forms of lymphoma and leukemia to try to relate to the symptoms. When my husband came home that evening I was sitting on the floor, my knees to my chest with a book of symptoms cradled in my arms. I was staring straight ahead. He knew instantly something was terribly wrong and sat down next to me. I said nothing for a few minutes and then I told him.

It took nearly a month after my bone marrow biopsy to receive the diagnosis from the University of Arizona Cancer Center in Tucson: LGL-leukemia, a rare form of chronic leukemia. It was a chronic condition that was expected to last forever, unless it escalated into an acute form which then could become terminal. For this reason, the physicians monitored my blood work every three months. Methotrexate was the recommended treatment, but I again rejected it. After I got the initial news, and allowed myself to wallow in pity for a few days (yes, that's absolutely normal), I began massive doses of Vitamin C and started emotional therapy by using Caroline Myss' and Louise Hay's books. My blood work stabilized and I expected to continue my therapies until the white count and lymph count gradually declined. They did. Twenty months later both were perfectly normal and I was well. That was more than seven years ago.

Hyperthyroidism

In the midst of the leukemia diagnosis, I began seeing a thickening in my neck - like a goiter appearing. I had noticed it in photos and thought I'd go once again to my holistic M.D. for her opinion. She sent me to an endocrinologist since I had a few other symptoms as well, where I was diagnosed with hyperthyroidism, a condition that over time can produce a goiter in the neck, irritability, heat intolerance, increased sweating, protruding eyes, and often tachycardia. After the initial visit and analyzing the results of my blood work, the endocrinologist was very eager to prescribe a pretty drastic but common treatment. She wanted the therapy done right away – actually by the following week. It consisted of giving me radioactive iodine, which would render my thyroid inactive. Thereafter, I'd take daily medication to replace the thyroxin my thyroid normally produced. The endocrinologist assured me the treatment was harmless, yet I couldn't be around children or pregnant women for 48 hours, among other incredible precautions. As you might guess, after more independent research and realizing I had years not days for this condition to affect my heart, I rejected her urgent manner and the radical treatment. My condition was not imminently critical and I ended up overcoming it with a simple therapy: tincture of iodine.

You Can Do It, Too

With each of these afflictions I was led to answers once I asked for help and surrendered. Because I was sometimes in shock and other times simply worn out from the condition, I learned to follow instead of always leading and I began to experience success. Not once, not twice, but many times. When reflecting on the process, I realized there were a number of common elements that occurred over and over. It was amazing that I was being directed, not to popular answers, but to the answers that were right for me and for my body. Had I not been open to receive, had interjected myself in a controlling way (my normal modus operandi) and taken this journey off track, I am positive I would have not have recovered.

During those twenty-some-years, while I was overcoming the virtual avalanche of health challenges, I found answers when I had been told none existed. With those outside-the-box solutions, I managed to heal without side effects. In fact, my body got stronger, more vibrant and healthier in the process. I am a woman who looks and acts much younger than her years, with energy to spare. Those characteristics are hard to demonstrate when one is in pain or otherwise very ill. It is simply impossible to look, feel and act great when you are suffering.

Today I watch people struggle needlessly with conditions they are told are chronic or incurable - but which are not. It breaks my heart to see these individuals become victims of a system that rejects other options outside their own and that intimidates patients into believing conventional medicine has the only answers. The result is these patients accept what they hear and give in. They give in to death or give in to damaging therapies that often do more harm than good.

In this book I will share a process, leading you to the perfect answers to heal holistically. The method of healing is called holistic healing, meaning to heal the whole. Although the elements of the methodology appear different for each person, the method can still be taught. You will learn not only the process I used, but can explore what a holistic healing journey looks and feels like - from a patient's perspective. You will also learn what to expect and will gain helpful hints to make your journey easier. The holistic healing I will describe is not a general one-size-fits-all program but rather is a customized process, complex in nature, which will be right for you. Best of all, you will come to realize additional benefits besides improved health that can be gained along the way: a greater sense of self-worth, more balance in your life, and an increased spiritual connection, which as you will come to know - may be the greatest gift of all. Even if you decide to make alternative methods only a complimentary part of the conventional treatments you are currently using, this book will be invaluable.

I am living proof answers exist. If I can find freedom from disease – many others can too. If I can heal on a deeper level –

many others can too. And, if I can be given guidance and direction to make both those things possible - many others can too. So, congratulations for reading this book. If you have been diagnosed with any condition you've been told has no cure or any condition you've been told is chronic - this is *your* book. If you're frustrated because you are aging too quickly, can't find good preventive advice, or the quality of your life seems to be slipping away while a doctor blames it on "age", this book will also be a blessing.

If you are one of the millions who experience a growing frustration with conventional medicine at some level, this book should provide hope because as people attempt to navigate the world of alternative medicine, many find it overwhelming and quit. They find too many options, with no one person to direct the entire process, and too little covered by medical insurance. People become fearful and rush back to a form of medicine that may not truly be right for them. They simply store away the frustration, disbelief, distrust, and disappointment they had for the conventional medicine system and return to blindly following their doctor's orders regardless of the consequences to their bodies.

One last thing. You need to understand that I am not anti-medicine. I believe in all the wonders of conventional medicine, if it is used judiciously. I don't believe in overuse, over testing, over prescribing or rushing into radical treatments when there are less invasive and less destructive methods available that could be tried first. I also don't believe M.D.'s have all the answers - for everything. There is a role for the patient, too. Personal responsibility should also be key. Yes, the health care system needs reform - but that reform starts with us.

This book will not prescribe. It will not tell you which vegetable to eat, which vitamin to take or which practitioner to see. Rather, it will show you how to find the perfect answers for you and help manage expectations as you move ahead.

I heard it once said that holistic healing is what we were truly intended to do, whether we were meant to die from our condition or not. I never understood the full concept of that statement until I experienced true, holistic healing for myself. Come with me now and you will see how to become well - if you are meant to be well - and how to heal, regardless.

It takes courage to launch a journey into the unknown. That is why I am giving you this roadmap. Use it with confidence and you will find a world of surprises, a better quality of life than you ever dreamed possible, and a form of healing that is profound.

SECTION ONE

Steps To Finding
The Perfect Answers
To Heal

Shatter Old Paradigms
Old Beliefs Aren't Always The Best Beliefs

T hroughout our lives our belief system is formed by what we observe and what we are told. As children, our parents were likely the major influence, although while growing up our peers and teachers also help shape the foundation of what we deem as true. The beliefs we hold have a lasting impact on our daily lives. They help form our attitudes about people and key situations but even more importantly, they help influence what we attract into our lives. "Money is the root of all evil." "Blood is thicker than water." "It's who you know." "Work hard and you will become a success. "These and other teachings can make the difference between affluence and poverty, success and failure and chronic illness and good health.

Looking At Your Body Differently

For the most part, we have been taught to ignore our body unless we are gauging its weight, assessing its beauty or attractiveness, or analyzing its function. When you look into the mirror what do you see? Do you define yourself by your weight or a physical flaw of some sort you always wished you could fix? Are you critical of your body? Do you experiment with diet after diet and help keep your cosmetic surgeon or local gym in business? Well, don't feel alone. Join the millions and millions of people, just like you, who believe their body is only physical, take it for granted, and probably miss or ignore its greatest gifts.

Let's start at the beginning and begin to reframe how we think about the incredible structure in which we live. When we first came into this world, each of us had only one thing with us - our body. This unique package, this miracle machine, was our first birthday gift; the one given to us by God, or if you prefer, a Higher Power. It is, without question, the most ingenious mechanism ever devised.

Just think about it - if we were living in a much more primitive society, our body would be our only tool for survival. Its instincts would lead us to nourishment and protect us from harm. We would nurture it by keeping it clean, grooming it and sheltering it from the elements. We would treat it with respect. Instead we were born in a much more sophisticated time, yet with all our education and worldliness we ignore the most important tool we were given for survival. Yes, even in this modern age - our body is a survival tool into which most of us have barely tapped.

I believe we would all agree that we take our body for granted. We push it to the limits, don't give it the right food, rarely give it the rest it needs, fill it full of drugs and chemicals to mask its normal reactions and rarely listen to the signals it gives us every day. The only time we pay attention to our physical selves is when we look into the mirror. And, then, it is generally in the form of an assessment: we are either too fat or too thin, we are getting wrinkles, our ears stick out, or there is some other flaw that we wish didn't exist. When we complain about how our body is beginning to break down, how it doesn't operate as well as it did when we were younger – it is always with a criticism, rarely a compliment. Yes, most of us take better care of our cars then we do with the machine in which we dwell.

For a change, let's consider our body from a different point of view. That's important because your body will be your partner in this healing journey. It will guide you and reflect the progress you are making along the way. But, before we get into the methodology, let's take a look at some of the wondrous achievements this body of ours accomplishes every day. Our bodies are pretty smart. For example, if we start to reach for something very hot and our body senses or feels the searing heat, our hand or arm instantly pulls back. We don't have to think about it or give it a conscious command - our bodies just do it automatically. If we walk along a road and a speeding car swerves too close, our bodies react, again, and we jump out of the way. This is automatic, too. We don't say, "Gee, that car is coming awfully close, I had better get out of the way." By then, of course, we'd be history. The reaction from our body happens within a split second - without any intellectual thought and without analyzing the situation. Our bodies help us survive.

Our body does a million other things for us in a twenty-four hour period that we don't realize, and routinely does dozens of things at once. We can be walking down the street with a friend while we are seeing and appreciating the surrounding scenery and at the same time hearing background noise, chewing and tasting gum, breathing and swallowing. All this is happening simultaneously while we're engrossed in conversation. Lest we forget, our body might also be digesting a late breakfast and fighting-off the possibility of a cold we were exposed to a couple of days before. All of this occurs a the same time. We don't consciously plan it and we don't think about it while it's happening. It is perfectly synchronized and spontaneous. It is totally orchestrated and managed without any conscious help.

It is really pretty amazing, when we take time to think about it. Just the routine stuff is a miracle, but what happens when we have an accident? Look at the healing properties our body then calls into action. When we receive a minor cut, blood comes rushing to the surface to purify the wound. That same blood seals the cut and helps it heal. Before long, the bleeding completely stops and within a day or two the skin has permanently closed shut. What could have become a scar is fading into a fine line that eventually disappears. We didn't think about that, it happened all by itself.

Our bodies also provide us with a built-in pharmacy. When all systems are working properly, we have the capability to manufacture internally all the drugs we'd ever need for anything. Our body produces adrenaline when we are under extreme stress and need extra energy or strength. We routinely fight off infection with our own form of antibiotics. We produce chemicals to aid sleep and can manufacture others to dull pain. Our bodies routinely produce whatever is required to fight bacteria, cancers and other foreign substances that pop up inside us all the time whether through some genetic quirk or by accident. Our system of healing is continual.

Our body also holds an enormous reserve of miraculous power into which we've not begun to tap. Some mystics, shamans, masters in martial arts, and paranormalists have managed extraordinary feats by tapping into the power of the very same body we were all given. They haven't been given any new gifts - they have just learned to access the ones we all have. They bend metal with their mind, levitate objects, walk on burning coals and break concrete blocks with a bare hand. Others elevate their body temperature so they are able to swim in freezing cold water for long distances with no protective clothing. Still others use their psychic powers and clairvoyant gifts to see the future and communicate with the spirit world. When tested to its farthest limits, our body is capable of unbelievable things; its potential is practically limitless.

Knowing all of this is possible and also recognizing that locked within this structure are resources we have yet begun to access, why should we ever doubt that our bodies have the capability to heal themselves? This body you were given is a miracle - your miracle. And, if you give it what it requires, listen to it and pay attention to its signals, your body will not let you down; it will be what guides you and eventually heals you completely.

In a later chapter, you will learn many more signals our bodies provide to help guide us to answers. Some of the simple, more obvious ones are pain - which usually indicates swelling, something out of alignment or a nerve issue, among other things. Coughs can mean something is in our lungs we need to expel or there is an irritation that is causing that reaction. Fever can mean our bodies are trying to eliminate an infection. Unfortunately in today's world we don't think about these symptoms as being signals to direct us to some other issue. Our doctors are trained to stop the signal - to eliminate the symptom. When we eliminate symptoms time-after-time, some fallout will ultimately occur.

Louise Hay, a noted author, publisher, and voice on alternative healing wrote a classic book titled *You Can Heal Your Life*, in which she lists the emotional root causes of almost any body issue. The emotional factor is a critical link in mind-body-spirit medicine. As you are probably aware, there are three levels in which we heal holistically: the physical, emotional and spiritual. Therefore, the emotional cannot be ignored. Her book is a terrific one, which I highly recommend. When something happens to your body, she believes and I concur, there is a way to interpret that signal as a sign for change or improvement in our lives. A knee injury, for example, represents pride and ego and could indicate stubbornness, the inability to bend, fear, inflexibility or that the individual will rarely give in. So, you can see how being aware of what is happening to your body can help you grow and improve as a person. She provides affirmations to help develop new thought patterns for each condition, one way to free-up blocked energy.

It is fun really, to look up such ailments, and they are always right on point. Her book is a very valuable tool for interpreting what our body is trying to tell us with whatever condition we face. It is a way to read our body for continued improvement and to learn what we need to clear emotionally, or to adjust attitudinally. A few more interesting examples include: ingrown toenail - worry and guilt about your right to move forward; lower back issues - fear of money or lack of financial support; nausea - fear, or rejecting an idea or experience and finally, nose bleeds - a need for recognition, feeling unrecognized and unnoticed, crying for love.[1] When multiple feelings are listed all rarely apply, therefore it is important to review the list and notice the one or ones that resonate with you. Sometimes being aware of the cause and beginning to make the changes helps stimulate the healing process.

In this chapter we just begin to scratch the surface of the role your body plays in your healing process. You won't, however, be able to fully appreciate its involvement until you begin to see this remarkable gift, your body, differently. Once you do, you will begin to have more gratitude and respect for the critical role it plays in your life.

Our Medical System Is The Best In The World

We have all been told the United States has produced the most magnificent system of medical care in the world and in the course of believing that, we continue to hold our doctors and the system that supports them in enormously high esteem. We believe our form of medicine is superior and ranks well above anything else - anywhere. Yet when we look at the facts, we find that it is not so.

In reviewing individual disease statistics and the progress we seem to be making, the data is confusing and sometimes conflicting, especially when one factors in population growth. However,

---

[1] Louise Hay, *You Can Heal Your Life* (Carlsbad:Hay House, 1999),176-221.

when we look at a simple little thing like life expectancy - it is easier to gain a more objective perspective.

According to a recent article in the Washington Post, "Americans are living longer than ever, but not as long as people in 41 other countries. For decades, the United States has been slipping in international rankings of life expectancy, as other countries improve health care, nutrition and lifestyles. Countries that surpass the U.S. include Japan and most of Europe, as well as Jordan, Guam and the Cayman Islands." The article then continues, "A baby born in the United States in 2004 will live an average of 77.9 years. That life expectancy ranks 42nd, down from 11th two decades earlier, according to international numbers provided by the Census Bureau and domestic numbers from the National Center for Health Statistics. Andorra, a tiny country in the Pyrenees mountains between France and Spain, had the longest life expectancy, at 83.5 years, according to the Census Bureau. It was followed by Japan, Macau, San Marino and Singapore. " [2]

This data gains greater perspective when one considers the enormous population and pollution challenges as well as the prevalent cigarette smoking in Japan, yet that country still ranks closer to the top of the list and greatly surpasses the U.S. There are other countries in Asia and Europe where cigarette smoking is also widely accepted that also rank higher than our country. So, why are we ranked so low? "The obesity rate in the U.S., rated on the highest in the world, is a factor as well as a relatively high

---

[2] Ohlemacher, Stephen. "*US Slipping in Life Expectancy Rankings.* " Washington Post (The Associated Press) 12 August 2007. <http://www.Washingtonpost.com>.

percentage of babies born in the U.S., who die before their first birthday compared with other industrialized nations." [2] Both pointing to a lack of personal responsibility (including prenatal care) and little focus on preventive healthcare by U.S. citizens. Could it be that we have been trained by a system that offers "quick fixes" administered *after* we become ill?

Some might argue the disparity is the result of having a percentage of our population not covered by health insurance. As compelling an argument as that might sound, most individuals who are not covered still seem to get treatment - even for routine care - at hospital emergency rooms where they are treated as charity cases and cannot be turned away. So, just because some people do not have health insurance does not mean they do not receive healthcare services.

There is another factor I happen to believe is relevant. People in other countries have more access to alternative forms of healthcare. Those methods are more open and more available and for that reason, perhaps these individuals simply make better personal choices in the care they select. There is also greater acceptance of alternative care in those countries which encourages their populations to look beyond allopathic methods for treatment. I just returned from Italy and France and saw exterior signs on every pharmacy I encountered that said "allopathic" on one side and "homeopathic" on the other. Inside I found both kinds of remedies. In the U.S., one has to go to a health food store, which for many lacks credibility, to find alternative remedies including homeopathic methods. In addition, many of these countries do not have a fast food restaurant on every corner.

If you are disturbed by the international comparison or find fault with my assessment, let's just stay focused on conventional medical care in the U.S. and let's take a look at how well that protects us.

Conventional Medicine Is The
Safest Route To Take

If we believe this is really true, let us first take a look at how our health care providers "first, do no harm", popularly believed part of the Hippocratic Oath traditionally taken by physicians. In their quest to "attack" or "kill" the germs, bacteria, viruses, cancers or other symptom causing invaders, physicians often ignore the body and the patient. This seek and destroy mission encourages many if not most doctors to jump to radical, invasive treatments right off the bat and prescribe highly toxic and damaging drugs to treat very minor ailments. Because they are in effect playing with fire, very often the patient gets burned. Yet, we remain loyal because we honestly believe medical doctors will take better care of us in the long run.

Well, consider the risk. According to an article in the Journal of the American Medical Association that analyzed patient care, the U.S. medical system is not as free of risk as we are led to believe and does great damage in the process of the practice of medicine. So if you are one of those who believe sticking with conventional medicine is the safest route, perhaps you should consider the following: According to several research studies in the last decade, including the aforementioned article, we find a total of 225,000 Americans per year die as a result of prescribed medical treatments. This is not disease caused deaths - it is treatment caused deaths. There are routinely 12,000 deaths per year due to unnecessary surgery, 7,000 deaths due to medication errors in hospitals, 20,000 deaths due to other hospital errors, 80,000 deaths due to infections contracted in hospitals and 106,000 deaths due to negative effects of drugs. All of these are annual numbers. Thus, America's healthcare-system's 225,000 induced mortalities are the third leading cause of death in the U.S., after heart disease and cancer.[3] Do we expect the medical community to be human and make mistakes? Sure. But, we also must acknowledge that the tools they are using are not always as effective as we might hope and are very often lethal. For that reason alone, I would always proceed with caution.

Knowing the statistics help us maintain our objectivity. More importantly, realizing the damaging effects that drugs, radiation and surgeries can cause helps us weigh more carefully the willingness to jump into treatments without thinking. It should also give us the courage to seek second opinions, consider other options and listen to our own good judgment in the process of deciding what medical treatment makes sense for us. Still, in the face of facts like these, our medical community still continues to be arrogant and dismissive of alternative options. There are an isolated number of physicians who will allow you to talk freely about alternative methods you may be using and some who even

---

[3] B Stanfield, "Is US Health Really The Best In The World?" *Journal of the American Medical Association, 284(4),* (2000, July 26), *483-485.*

11

encourage complimentary options, but for the most part medical physicians are threatened by a trend toward alternatives in which they have not been trained and cannot control.

As a healthcare consumer, being educated is critical to keep from misplacing your trust. Take cancer patients for example. According to Deepak Chopra, M.D., in *Ageless Body Timeless Mind*, if cancer patients were really aware of the facts regarding this disease, there might be a major shift away from conventional medicine for treatment. Instead, there appears to be a prevalent belief that medicine has come a long way in curing cancer. People believe that whatever treatment is given today is better than the condition they have. That belief is not based on fact. The age-adjusted death rate from cancer has not changed in fifty years. Modern treatments do not prolong life overall even though the perception exists that cancer patients are living longer than they did in the past because of early detection.[4] Doctors today are doing more to fight cancer but not necessarily getting better results - and they are doing a lot of unnecessary damage to our bodies in the process.

Conventional Medicine Is The Only Way To Go

If this is true, why are so many brilliant, high-profile physicians are becoming alternative advocates? It is interesting to note that for more than twenty years highly respected medical profes-

---

[4] Deepak Chopra, M.D., *Ageless Body Timeless Mind* (New York: Harmony Books, 1993), 250.

sionals have been expanding their practices in the medical field to include holistic and alternative methods. Many have completely walked away from allopathic medicine. The most popular and most celebrated spokespersons in the world of alternative or complimentary healthcare were all allopathically trained: Deepak Chopra, M.D., the brilliant endocrinologist who also taught at Tufts University and Boston University Schools of Medicine; Andrew Weil, M.D., a graduate of the Harvard Medical School and was a former researcher in Ethno pharmacology at Harvard; Christiane Northrup M.D., trained at Dartmouth Medical School and Tufts New England Medical Center and is board certified in obstetrics and gynecology; Larry Dossey, M.D., former Chief of Staff of Humana Medical City Dallas; Bernie Seigel, M.D., a gifted surgeon who also taught at Yale University; O. Carl Simonton, M.D., a former radiation oncologist and Mehmet Oz, a Harvard educated Professor of Cardiac Surgery at Columbia University, renowned heart surgeon and founder of the Complementary Medicine Program at New York Presbyterian Hospital. These brilliant minds and many more just like them, all promote options that tell us conventional medicine does not do everything well and that other answers exist outside the confines of that modality's rigid doctrine. These individuals have huge followings, sell millions of books and tapes, and have become celebrities in their own right.

When I try to name popular allopathic "voices" I can think of only one: Dr. Dean Edel, popular radio commentator, who appears to me still to be a skeptic regarding most alternative methods. When you weigh the dollars spent attending workshops and seminars, buying books and tapes and watching TV appearances of the alternative voices versus the strictly allopathic messengers, it seems to me the more popular are those embracing available alternative options.

In local communities doctors are leaving their profession every day to find careers in a field that is certainly not as lucrative but ultimately more rewarding - serving people through holistic or alternative means. My cardiologist recently left her practice to become a homeopathic physician. My acupuncturist is a former medical anesthesiologist. My naturopath was trained as a registered nurse. Look around and you will see others who have not made a total switch, yet are becoming more open to the possibilities that exist elsewhere. I am sure each of you is aware of a medical professional or two who has also defected to holistic medical practices.

Your Doctor Knows Best

With the advent of conventional medicine less than two hundred years ago and more advanced scientific medicine less than a hundred years ago, we have still been conditioned to believe our doctors know everything about healthcare and healing. Over time, they began to believe it, too. Today we find that we've devoted ourselves to a standard of care that is good but not great, that doesn't include preventive maintenance or education, and that ignores personal responsibility. It is no surprise we are not as healthy as we think we are and there are many reasons for this. Our doctors do not understand nutrition, we are not encouraged to pay attention to our total bodies, and we are given few tools to combat stress. Our country has produced obese children and adults as well as a horribly sedentary population that is living on foods full of calories, and stripped of nutrients. We are over-stressed and getting cancer more frequently than ever before in our history, fighting world-wide viruses drugs cannot cure, and seeing cases of Alzheimer's and autism skyrocket.

Make no mistake, the role of the physician has changed: from friendly family doctors who were good neighbors, made house calls, cared about our families and listened to our "stories" - to physicians who transformed themselves into intimidating fig-ures with impressive offices, hours that work for them and very few minutes to spare for patients. During this metamorphosis in which we changed from loving them to being intimidated by them, we helped create the monster that is now dictating our care. We are partially to blame.

It's true, over the years our doctors have given us less and less time to explain what was going on in our lives so they could more clearly see what was going on with our bodies, but then we also didn't demand it. The result: physicians diagnosing in a va-cuum, within a system that's simply out of whack. Soon we began to believe what we had to say didn't matter and they believed it, too. Today, our physicians actually believe we know very little - they especially ignore and dismiss what women and seniors have to say. Our symptoms are minimized and if we have multiple symptoms, they are often written-off as psychosomatic or over-blown. No wonder the "cures" they provide rarely do anything but attack the presenting, most pressing "symptom" and do nothing to get to the root cause of the condition. In all fairness, sharing the blame should also include today's medical schools, which rein-force the same ideology and nurture the beast.

15

Dr. Christiane Northrup, M.D., a prominent author and physician who advocates holistic healing, has an interesting perspective about cures. She writes that a cure will relieve your symptoms but healing does a more thorough job with the underlying problem that's causing those symptoms. She states that a cure is temporary, like a painkiller or a laxative, or in more drastic cases, a mastectomy or hysterectomy. With cures, you may feel better at first. Yet, in almost every case she's seen, the cure is temporary because cures don't get to the heart of the matter; cancers return in another form or a weak body continues to contract other conditions. Healing, however, almost always lasts because healings happen from the inside out and affect the total body.[5]

Most medical professionals are not well equipped to help in the true healing process. They look at symptoms, treat symptoms and don't have the time or inclination to be bothered with the ancillary matters that affect your total body and thereby ultimate health. This is where holistic practitioners are different and why their processes may work better for some conditions. They are specialists in evaluating the whole body for answers. For a point of clarity, an M.D. can also be a holistic provider although they are few and far between. In the greater Phoenix Metro area, which is the fifth largest city in the United States, although there may be a few more, I know of only a handful.

---

[5] Christiane Northrup, M.D., "*How to Create a Health Miracle In Your Life.*" A promotional flier article: 1997, 15.

Always Follow Your Doctor's Orders

Instead of turning all your power over to the physician sitting in front of you, remember you actually have choices. Your power comes when you exercise your choices and speak up when needed. For example, there is a time to choose conventional medicine and a time to choose something else - or nothing at all. They key is to know when to do what.

Andrew Weil, M.D., whom as I mentioned earlier was educated at Harvard and is an articulate and authoritative voice for alternative healing, acknowledges that allopathic medicine does not have all the answers. He lists in his book *Spontaneous Healing,* what you can expect from conventional medicine and what you cannot. The <u>can</u> list includes: managing trauma better than any other system of medicine, diagnosing and treating medical and surgical emergencies, treating acute bacterial infections with antibiotics, treating some parasitic and fungal infections, preventing many infectious diseases by immunization, diagnosing complex medical problems, replacing damaged hips and knees, getting good results with cosmetic and reconstructive surgery, and diagnosing and correcting hormonal deficiencies.

Dr. Weil continues that allopathic medicine <u>cannot</u>: adequately treat viral infections, cure most chronic degenerative diseases, effectively manage most kinds of mental illness, cure most forms of allergy or auto immune disease, effectively manage psychosomatic illnesses, or cure most forms of cancer.[6]

---

[6] Andrew Weil, M.D., *Spontaneous Healing* (New York: Alfred A. Knopf, Inc., 1995), 225-226.

Most objective physicians should agree with this list. I have a couple of exceptions, however. The jury is still out, as far as I'm concerned, whether conventional medicine does such a great job correcting hormonal deficiencies in women - as we all know from the conflicting philosophies surrounding hormone replacement therapy. I am also doubtful about their ability to diagnose complex medical problems that are stress related or that stem from conditions such as candida albicans, since they rarely acknowledge this condition as potentially serious. Finally, there are alternative treatments for fungal and parasitic infections that are just as effective and carry fewer side effects than those prescribed by conventional medicine. Dr. Weil, I believe, is being generous to his colleagues. Other than those whom I feel compelled to refute, I believe his list is right on the money. So, if you have a chance, copy this list and post it somewhere to remind you.

Once you become more aware of the limitations of your physician, you become smarter about how much you trust and how much power you turn over. Running to a doctor for many of the things they do not manage successfully is a waste of time and money, and could ultimately result in needless damage to your body in the process.

Medical practitioners are willing to admit their vulnerability regarding certain conditions and illnesses among themselves; however, dialogue on this topic doesn't always extend to the patient. In the last 20 years, as I mentioned earlier, there have been a number of prominent medical doctors who have been more open and candid about the weaknesses of their profession and are willing to share that knowledge with the rest of us. Those physicians are still M.D.'s but have augmented their medical practices with other non-conventional treatment protocols. They are attempting to overcome the inherent limitations of their field. They all expound holistic healing and by expanding what these physicians, and many others, offer to their patients they have tried to improve on the voids of their primary medical training.

More books are being daily published by medical doctors who, in trying to move their patients to wellness, have reached beyond conventional medicine. Some of these physicians urge patients to stick with allopathic care and supplement their healing ritual with other means, while others encourage patients to utilize primarily alternative methods. They espouse holistic healing and by expanding what these physicians, and many others, offer to their patients, they try to improve the shortcomings in their previous medical training.

Regardless which road you choose, you must realize that choices do exist and you have the power to make those choices. For those of you unfamiliar with options outside conventional medicine, there is a wide array of choices. In the Addendum to this book I list the most popular. There is a world of options when you really look around.

Now, for those of you who prefer to function totally outside the typical medical community, I caution you to also maintain some kind of ongoing relationship with a conventional medical professional who can offer periodic, scientific diagnostic help. Of all the wonders modern medicine has accomplished, none is more amazing than the advances that have been made in diagnosing illness: the sophisticated lab techniques for analyzing our blood and urine, biopsy tests and DNA tests, and the remarkable inroads being made in genetic research. Amazing tools like CAT-scans and MRIs look into our tissue and bone to reveal secrets we never imagined. Every day, there are more and more phenomenal inventions available to identify and analyze our bodies. Early diagnosis is not only important – it is critical to a long life and a good quality of life. It is important to know what you must overcome.

A simple rule of thumb to remember is if you have an acute condition with a very, very short window of opportunity for treatment - like hours, days or weeks - you will probably need to begin with conventional medical intervention. If a longer window of opportunity exists – you will have time for alternative methods, which offer fewer side effects and very often a more complete healing experience.

Totally Believe
What Your Doctor Tells You

The worst thing our medical practitioners do to us is program our defeat. When a doctor tells you that you will have to live with a condition forever or that you might not live very long at all – it has serious impact. When words like that are spoken something very powerful occurs. If you believe what is said, it zaps you of any remaining control and strength, robs you of your self-confidence and creates a placebo-in-reverse effect. A powerful and damaging dynamic is created by physicians who overstep their field of knowledge by attempting to fortune-tell their patient's future.

Doctors don't realize the damage they can do. The problem lies not so much in delivering the diagnosis, but rather how they actually deliver the prognosis. Patients are too often told; "There is no cure for this condition." "All we can do is treat the symptoms - the condition will not go away." "You will just have to live with it." "There is nothing more that can be done." - or even more shocking, "You only have three to six months to live."

There are other, more truthful options. It is perfectly fine for doctors to deliver their interpretation of fact, but they should do so with hope. Simply adding the caveat that a patient "doesn't have to be one of the statistics" is not being dishonest - instead it keeps hope alive. A physician would be even more truthful if he or she said, "We don't have a good track record with this disease our odds offer only a 50 percent survival rate. But, you don't have to be one of those statistics, you can look elsewhere." Or, they could simply say, "I am not able to help you, however, help could exist in another form of treatment." These approaches not only keep hope alive but are also the truth.

When a patient who is vulnerable and is already fearful of a bad diagnosis hears a prognosis of doom, it can become a self-fulfilling prophecy or worse - it can become a hex. We have all heard of the placebo response, with patients showing improvement if they simply believe they are taking something that will help them. Well, that same response can work in reverse. The power of the mind is astounding; people can believe there is no hope if a negative message is delivered by someone they trust.

In reading through a number of articles and papers by Dr. Howard Brody Co-Author of *The Placebo Response* and Professor of Family Medicine and Philosophy at Michigan State University, I was able to ascertain that a positive placebo response occurs when three factors are optimally present: the meaning of the illness experience for the patient is altered in a positive manner; the patient is supported by a caring group; and the patient's sense of mastery and control over the illness is enhanced. It became clear to me that a physician can strip a patient of two or three of these factors with a poorly worded prognosis.

If a physician has made an absolute statement with the medical diagnosis or prognosis to you, without offering any hope at all, a behavioral command has been established. This then becomes the predominant mind-set for everyone surrounding you. You believe it, your doctor believes it, all who treat you believe it and your family and friends believe it, therefore, that prognosis is precisely what occurs.

Sometimes your doctor doesn't have to say anything at all, except name the disease. Today, there isn't much of a discussion about the eventual outcome once HIV-AIDS and even some forms of cancer are diagnosed, but there should be. We have all been conditioned to believe having HIV-AIDS means a certain, eventual death sentence. The fact exists that conventional, allopathic medicine has no known cure; however, by using other measures, patients can go on to live full productive lives. Unfortunately, not enough people look past the scientific, medical model to see if hope exists through other methods. They expect to die and that's exactly what they do.

Follow Your Physician's Timeline, Too

There is yet another habit existing in the medical profession which does irreparable harm. That is the habit of rushing one into treatment whether or not it is needed immediately. Let me give you an example. After being diagnosed with LGL-leukemia, part of my mission was to identify other secondary infections, which might be occurring in my body that could also affect the rise in my lymph count. This strategy was pointed out to me by a wise holistic practitioner, Dr. Hugh Riorden, who operated an alternative focused cancer research and treatment center in Wichita, Kansas. Dr. Riorden said to me, while I was seated next to him at a dinner, "I'd be curious, if I were you, about why your lymphocyte count is so high." I, of course, thought that was all just part of having the kind of leukemia with which I had been diagnosed."Lymphocytes fight low grade infections," Riorden continued. At that point, it didn't take long for me to figure out that if my immune system was busy fighting off a low-grade infection it certainly couldn't focus on fighting my leukemia. So, if I could get rid of these secondary conditions, it might speed-up my healing.

In the process of identifying a number of issues my body had that could distract my immune system, including Epstein-Barr, H-pylori and parasites - another condition surfaced. My throat had become swollen at the base of the neck and it was becoming extremely tender. Actually, the condition was represented by the thickening I had first noticed in recent photographs of me, which you may remember I recounted in the events surrounding my hyperthyroid diagnosis. I felt racy even though I was tired and seemed to have flashes of being warmer at night than my normal menopausal symptoms. In blood work I had taken, my thyroid reading was also slightly elevated, so I made the appointment with an endocrinologist.

The doctor selected was a charming woman. She was very patient and kind and quite interested in my leukemia and what I was doing to treat myself so successfully since I was not getting regular medical treatment for my condition. She also stated that since she only knew about the methods in which she was trained, she couldn't render an opinion. I thought her honesty was refreshing and thought she would be more flexible in her approach.

After she read the results of the blood work taken in her office, she confirmed hyperthyroidism. She also cautioned me that a weakening of the heart was the downside risk to leaving this condition untreated for a long period of time and encouraged an immediate procedure which involved destroying my thyroid's ability to function. I asked for clarification of the phrase "long period of time". "Are we talking weeks and months or are we talking years before ultimate risk?" I queried. She clarified her reference by saying she meant many years of being left untreated but still stressed the need for this drastic treatment using radioactive iodine to destroy the function of my thyroid. Following that destructive process, I would be given a daily pill for the rest of my life to replace the thyroid hormone.

When I asked her why I would want to put radioactive material in my body while I had this leukemia, she assured me the radioactive material was harmless. In the next breath, she said. "When we administer the dose to destroy the thyroid function, you will be asked to sleep alone for 48 hours; you should not share any eating or drinking utensils with others and should not be around pregnant women or small children. The danger to others during this period is that their thyroid, too, might also become dysfunctional." This told me the procedure was hardly harmless.

She hoped we could schedule a preliminary radioactive test that afternoon and begin the treatment a few days later.

She was quite firm in everything she said and I had little time to even react, let alone do research on my own. This doctor was pushing me into a test and the follow-up treatment much too quickly. I am a strong willed, outspoken person but even I was intimidated by her manner. As she had asked, I scheduled my test for a week from that day at the front desk then left. A day or two later I called her office and cancelled the test. I told them I'd call later to reschedule, but never did.

Research from the Internet on my own confirmed I had a few of the common symptoms of hyperthyroidism but I had no swollen fingers, nail problems, insomnia, elevated pulse or blood pressure, etc. Plus, what symptoms I had were mild. I also called my previous doctor and found my thyroid test was only slightly elevated two weeks earlier. A holistic physician recommended a simpler procedure and clearly one less invasive. I applied a small amount of iodine to my forearm measuring the length of time it took to absorb - an alternative method for determining any iodine deficiency exists, which for some is the cause of hyperthyroidism. The result? I improved without radical radioactive iodine destroying my thyroid. Ironically, a few weeks later, I asked my regular physician to do a thyroid test to see how it was doing. This time, my thyroid tested low.

Being too quick to jump into any radical treatment that has damaging side effects is never smart. Doing a little research, seeking a second opinion and waiting until you are more comfortable with the procedure is always the wisest choice.

If you feel rushed by the scheduling of tests or treatments, you have the power to take the prescription and not fill it right away. You also have the power to schedule the test and then cancel or reschedule it. And, you have the power to question why something appears to be so urgent. You are in control and you must realize there may be other reasons doctors push treatment besides the imminent risk to the patient. For some physicians, that reason could be as simple as increased monthly revenues.

Don't Be Too Forceful Or Challenge Your Doctor

You have the right to be in control when it comes to anything that impacts your body. In case you doubt the amount of control you truly have, consider this. Ultimate control lies in the amount of information one possesses. Now, although doctors have medical studies, technical knowledge of the workings of the body and knowledge of the reactions and interactions of drugs, they don't know you. You, on the other hand, have knowledge of your body: how it feels, what it is doing on a day-to-day basis, what stresses have occurred or are occurring in your life that could cause or exacerbate a condition and all the details of your lifestyle, such as what you eat and drink and how, or even if, you relax. You also know your emotional make-up and what might have occurred in early years that could have some underlying effect on your life and health today. Finally, you understand the depth or lack of depth in your spirituality; how much faith you have and how much hope you have.

In a nutshell, you know yourself better than anyone else - including your doctor. That is why this process should be a partnership and why the path to getting well should take into account everything about you. The treatment should be holistic.

So, think of your relationship with your doctor this way. Your doctor can diagnose, recommend, write prescriptions and schedule future appointments. But, if you are uncertain or uncomfortable with what he or she has to say, you have the power and personal responsibility to seek another opinion, ignore the recommendation, not fill the prescription, or to cancel future appointments. Nobody can make you do anything you don't want to do. Until you are comfortable and until you have all the information you need, you don't have to do anything at all.

If You Can't Prove It Scientifically – It Isn't Valid

Conventional medicine is stuck on statistics; if there hasn't been a double blind study done and if you can't measure it – it can't possibly work. Well, who can measure faith, for example? Who can measure personal responsibility? Who can measure diligence? All three make a huge difference in a person's health or healing approach even though all three are relatively immeasurable by themselves. If you take two identical individuals with the same basic illness, the same basic education and grades, and the same basic health history, it will always be the one with the greater faith, the personal responsibility, the diligence - or all three that will get well quicker than the other. Then, of course, there is the role of the belief system - not considered a significant treatment tool but proven time and time again to be a factor in studies where placebos and their reverse effect are proven reactions. These scientific studies focus on the drug or procedure and rarely dissect the placebo or its opposite response, itself, to understand how the belief system drives the result.

Most everyone has heard of the placebo effect but the reverse, as I mentioned earlier, also has a name. The nocebo response is when a drug-trial subject's symptoms are worsened by the administration of an inert or dummy (simulator) treatment called a placebo. Since the placebo would have contained no chemical or agent that could possibly have caused any of the observed worsening of the subject's symptoms or side-effects, the change for the worse must be due to some subject-internal factor. The term itself was coined in 1961 by Walter Kennedy and the word was selected because it is the opposite Latin word to placebo "I shall please" and means "I shall harm".[7] Both responses happen over-and-over in clinical studies and are acknowledged but otherwise virtually ignored.

If we look carefully at alternative results versus the results achieved by allopathic means, we find that although the factors mentioned above may not be scientifically measured, they do exist and are factored as key elements in most alternative protocols. The belief system can be linked to affirmations and visualization, which help our subconscious form or change an existing belief system into something different. Faith is an absolute - both through the power of prayer and the existence of a

---

[7] Wikipedia Free Online Encyclopedia, http://en.wikipedia.org/wiki /Nocebo

positive outlook in general. Faith, overall, ensures a belief that a positive result will occur, which is certainly part of the alternative mix. Spirituality then comes into play by practicing love to eliminate destructive negative emotions from our bodies and by forgiv-forgiving, which is very healing in and of itself. Diligence and personal responsibility relate totally to how one manages his or her lifestyle. These can include how people apply nutrition, use supplements, reduce stress, and the effect of routine habits like getting enough sleep, exercise, and even meditation, to help recover. The medical community acknowledges many of these factors but doesn't bestow on them the same level of importance as drug therapy, radiation or surgery, alone. The alternative elements recounted are simply not taken seriously enough by conventional doctors. Because physicians are untrained in many of these factors, they are unable to even remotely assess their presence in a patient's life.

There is a reason why it is very difficult to measure a holistic healing program scientifically - and probably why it is never done. True holistic healing is a customized mix for each individual's body and is based on the information gathered from lengthy discussions with the patient. There is no one formula and no one-size-fits-all, because we are each unique. The most effective solutions are always comprehensive approaches influenced by myriad factors. Make sense? Conversely, the scientific studies are typically focused on one condition and utilize one drug or one surgical or medical procedure in a universal body of people who appear similar. Comparing the two is like comparing a solo flute to an orchestra.

Still, we find arrogance and intolerance in the medical community regarding most alternative options evidenced by Dr. George Lundberg, editor of the Journal of the American Medical Association who was quoted by the British Medical Journal as saying "There is no 'alternative medicine,' only scientifically proven medicine." He continued, "In God we trust; all others must have data," quoting his colleague Dr. Claude Organ, editor of the Archives of Surgery.[8]

Let's look again at the scientific studies and try to dissect the process. Let's say in a good result, patients using the tested drug improved (to some degree) 80 percent of the time. The words to focus on are "to some degree" because every person is different and some have incredible results while others have only slight - yet all in the group that get better; improve. So, the degree is often a factor. In some studies, of course, the method rids the patient of the condition totally but rarely without a price and there is no guarantee it won't return, which is why doctors often continue with routine follow-ups - sometimes for years. In addition, 20 percent still did not improve at all. Who is to say which percent you will fall into - the group who didn't improve, those who improved only slightly, those who improved moderately or those who improved greatly? When you factor all that into the equation the odds change from 80/20 to something much less if you are looking for a total recovery.

Then there is the side-effect issue. Every drug known to man produces some sort of side effect. For a drug to work it will either

---

[8] *British Medical Journal* - FMJ1009, 317:1038 (21 November, 1999).

do the job of your immune system, cause your immune system to stop working, or it will affect the function of your liver or kidneys, two key organs that are generally part of the detox process of the body. Those effects are guaranteed. Some will have even more dramatic consequences. The reason is that no two people will react the same is that while some body types react one way, others whose bodies absorb or process differently will react yet another. Some have more fragile immune systems, some have more vulnerable livers and kidneys, and others are more chemically sensitive overall.

What about those who got well without the drug? What doctors don't share with their patients is that there were some patients in the clinical trials who got the placebo and who still improved. The power of our belief system is again one of those things medicine cannot quantify but it extremely powerful. The point being, everything that involves our bodies is not projectable to the masses nor is it certain for each individual. Results are totally dependent upon the person's own body chemistry, history, lifestyle and belief system - which conventional medicine doesn't thoroughly consider.

Instead of a formula treatment - always with a risk factor attached - I personally choose to have a customized program that happens to work perfectly for my body. Even though I'm not a statistically valid result - I happen to like having been a successful anecdote over and over again.

Related to anecdotal results, medical doctors will tell you that these results are singular and random, and therefore don't count. Yet, when you analyze their process it is quite bizarre and not uniform at all. In building their studies, they look for a consis-

tent group to test and then consider the results of that test absolutely valid. But, by thinking the test groups selected were
consistently constructed is invalid in the first place. Take a look
around you; it is pretty difficult to put any of us into groups where
there is a total consistency – where individuality is not an enormous factor. So, let's say, they test a group of diabetics. They pick
people of a certain age who have the same type of diabetes and
who exhibit similar symptoms (as they previously defined). Out
of those 100 individuals no two are even close to being the same
person. They are different in terms of body type. For example,
some are ectomorphs, others are endomorphs and still others me-
somorphs. Those three body types don't function nearly the same.
Also consider other factors such as the fact that some people live
with more stress than others, some have genetic predispositions
others don't have, and still others have lifestyle habits that are
consistently destructive. These modifying factors are why the
people conducting these studies will *average* the amount of improvement in the group by the particular drug or surgical method
being tested. Everybody in the test group will react differently.
One will improve but have side effect A. The other will improve
slightly more and have side effect B and so on. By the time we
consider the side effects suffered balanced by the results we'd
have a totally different picture. Having something scientifically
proven sounds impressive, but when one starts to dissect the data
with all the resulting questions it appears less and less absolute.

Well, I am somewhat jaded in my opinion but a physician
will never tell you the odds are you will totally recover, have no
side effects and become healthier overall in the end. So I'm not a

scientific study fan and believe all that really matters is what works for you.

Thoughts to Consider

Our bodies protect us routinely, day-after-day without any conscious thought from us. Of course, they can also help us heal.

The potential of the human body is astounding. It might be interesting to tap into a little of that so you can reach wellness faster.

Our bodies communicate with us in many ways so slow down and pay attention to what yours is trying to tell you.

Steps to Take

Don't jump into radical treatments with damaging side effects unless you have done research, sought a second opinion or waited until you are totally comfortable with the procedure.

Remember what allopathic medicine does well and doesn't do well. Keep a list on where it can be easily referenced when you need to seek help.

You can agree with your diagnosis but you don't have to agree with your prognosis

Be a healthcare consumer.

Don't be one of the patients who is only trying to please your doctor.
Begin to please yourself

Become an active partner with your doctor. You know more about your body and lifestyle than anyone else.

Don't take your body for granted. Appreciate what it does for you and give it what it needs to run efficiently and effectively.

Treat your body with respect; it was your first birthday gift.

Begin to notice the signals your body sends.

Buy Louise Hay's book - *You Can Heal Your Life* - begin to relate your illnesses and accidents to messages your body is sending.

Don't be intimidated by those who use scientific studies to justify the absolute credibility of a drug or procedure.

Focus On The Right Thing
You Asked For It - But
You Got Something Else

R egardless of what condition you have and regardless of what you've been told about it, answers do exist to help you recover. The holistic process that will make your recovery a reality begins with a first step. It is the most important step since it deals with your intention - what you intend to achieve. If your goal is wrong the result will be wrong. You would be surprised how many people get messed up on this initial step although it seems so obvious. Initially the first step consists of three parts with which to deal: to become determined, to ask and to focus your intention on the right thing.

In this chapter I'll help you formulate the right frame of mind and help you become more acutely focused. Of course, the circumstances or motivation that brought you to this point will be unique with each of you. It could be that you're sick and tired of being sick and tired. Others might be fed up with all the drugs they're taking and believe there must be a better way. Maybe you have lost faith in your doctor and conventional medicine because they haven't been able to provide answers to really help you improve. Or, you could have a pressing reason for really wanting to get well - a new love, a first grandchild, or a passion in life you want to experience. Regardless your motivation - this is the process I used with great success.

First, Become Determined

Becoming determined is very different from simply wanting or hoping. Being bound and determined, digging in or being hell-bent are all ways to describe that strong, resolute, unwavering feeling you get when you know exactly where you are headed and don't intend to let anything or anybody get in your way. This determination is not an intellectual whim. It is a very deep feeling that you feel throughout your body. It is a commitment - a soul-felt promise. We all have felt determination at one time or another. Maybe it was as a child when we demanded from our little playmate with all the internal strength we could muster, "I don't care what you say, I *can climb that tree*." And, you did it. Or, as a teen when we practiced and practiced to try out for the sports team and finally made it. Or, as an adult, when we struggled through 18-hour days and put our life savings into our very own business that ultimately became a success.

When I hold healing workshops about finding the path to wellness, one of the first exercises I ask individuals to do is to identify a time in each of their lives when they had complete resolve to make something happen - and then did it. A time when they didn't let anything or anybody get in their way. I ask them to write a sentence or two describing that experience and then to remember that feeling of determination. That is the feeling I want you to capture once again.

You don't need to hold on to that feeling every moment throughout your journey in order to anchor the intent - but initially, that same determination must be present while you state your intention. You must be able to draw on that feeling if you ever think about quitting.

Ask For What You Want

Many of you reading this book have probably read *The Secret*, one of the best selling books in the last 20-years, about how to manifest what you want in your life. Or maybe you saw the video. The message provided is quite simple: Ask - Believe - Receive. Well, they communicated it right, the process works but in finding wellness there are a few more steps, including this one. Receiving rarely happens without some action from you - and what form that takes is not something you can anticipate in advance. Just be prepared because asking is the first part - then when the answer is delivered, your participation will likely be necessary to make it work.

I spoke my intention almost automatically and without realizing the power of my words as I left my rheumatologist's office in the early 80's. He had recommended I take a mild form of chemotherapy, Methotrexate, for my rheumatoid arthritis. This was just part of the natural progression of his treatment since my condition had not really improved even though my meds kept getting stronger. I was impatient with my life, this illness and was becoming more and more discouraged with conventional medicine.

After I told the doctor I didn't think I would try the newest drug, my husband and I proceeded to the car. That's when I said, "I don't think God wants me to suffer like this." I continued defiantly, "I know there are answers out there somewhere – and I intend to find them." I made the statement out loud and I meant with all my heart.

When my husband asked, "Well, what are you going to do, now?" I replied, " I don't know. I don't have a clue – but it isn't going to be this (Methotrexate)."

Being a problem solver by nature this approach really fit for me. Every problem had a solution and because I knew God had created a magnificent, wondrous and complex universe that we are only beginning to understand – of course there would be answers to help me. It made perfect sense.

Whatever you say in stating your intention has to make sense to you, too. So, you may want to state, "I intend to get well - whatever it takes." Or, "I will do whatever I have to do, go wherever I have to go or see whomever I have to see - in order to find wellness." You will begin to get the idea.

Once you find a statement that fits for you – state it out loud and deliver it firmly, absolutely and from your heart. God will hear you. The Universe will hear you and your body will hear you. Then, let it go and have faith. You don't need to say it over and over like an affirmation, if you totally believe the statement you are making. Then the answers to bring wellness into your life will be delivered to you – in the perfect order and at the perfect time. It is natural to worry that you weren't heard and doubt this will work but don't let fear creep into the picture. The first time any form of answer is delivered to you - and it will come within a relatively short period of time - then you will know you have ab-solutely been heard. At that point, just go with what comes. The first signal you get, or whatever happens will prove the Universe is now in charge.

Next, Focus On The Right Thing

I don't recall where I first heard the theory "what you focus on expands" but the first time I heard it was like remembering something I always knew. It may have been in a book or a tape by Dr. Wayne Dyer or Deepak Chopra but wherever it was, it stuck. After, I noticed that, when I placed my attention on something I could actually watch it grow – or more realistically become more important in my life. For example, when I started my manuscript, all of a sudden books, book reviews and authors started popping up all over the place. People started talking to me about writing and publishing. I was thrown into new groups - all of which seemed to be filled with authors. The part of my life I had focused on started to magnify.

You can try it yourself. If you are married to a partner who is a mixture of truly wonderful traits and a few irritating ones, notice where you are placing your focus. If you continually rivet your attention to the little imperfections, you will become more irri-tated and your relationship will evolve into something less than blissful. Pretty soon those imperfections will be the only things you begin to see. Every time one of those little annoying habits reappears, the negative image you have locked-in your mind about your mate is reconfirmed. Your reaction to the irritations becomes stronger and stronger and soon the wonderful things he or she does doesn't carry near as much weight as the "there he or she goes again" irritations. Each negative experience builds on the last negative experience until you have a mountain of episodes that begin to drive you crazy. Change your focus and your relationship will also change.

The same theory applies to your healing journey. Before you begin – you have to know where you are going. It is a matter of clear focus.

Let me tell you a story about a dear friend of mine, Gladys Taylor McGarey, M.D.(H), cofounder of the American Holistic Medical Association and a gifted physician, who has consistently helped her patients heal from a variety of illnesses during the more than sixty years she practiced medicine. A number of years ago, when Dr. Gladys and I met, I shared with her the journey I had taken to find wellness. She was delighted with my story, gave me my routine physical and encouraged me to keep doing exactly what I had been doing. Then she told me about two women patients she had treated - both with lupus.

She said one woman had dramatic results, just like I did. The second was a totally different story. As hard as she tried, Dr. Gladys could not help this woman recover. One day Dr. Gladys and the unsuccessful woman were leaving the office at the same time. They both walked to the parking lot and parted to go to their respective cars. Dr. Gladys remembered something she wanted to tell the woman and as she turned to call to her, she stopped dead in her tracks. The woman had the word LUPUS spelled on her license plate.

Here was a person who totally identified with her disease. She had not only accepted it, she was living it. Now Dr. Gladys knew why this woman had been unable to find total healing.

It doesn't matter what the reason this woman had for submerging herself in her disease - maybe it was to give her something to talk about with other people because she felt uninteresting as a person. Maybe it was because she didn't have much of a life, herself, and this gave her something to think about all day. The fact remained - this person needed to change her focus.

That change is tough for some people. It is tough for victims who want to blame everything outside themselves for all their problems. It is tough for people who have low self-esteem and don't believe their lives are worth battling for. It is also tough for people who receive more attention from others because of their condition than ever before - and, frankly, enjoy it.

In order to get well you must make a conscious effort to focus on wellness. Because of that, you will have a better chance at getting over this hurdle in your life and finding a new ways to approach your healing. It is perfectly fine to be realistic about where you are today, health-wise, but in addition, have a clear picture of where you intend to be tomorrow.

There's one final trap some people fall into, not playing the "name game" and denying the existence of their disease or condition. That, quite honestly, is not considered positive thinking – it is, instead, counter productive.

Here's an example. Amanda had chronic fatigue syndrome. She looked tired, worn and it was apparent to everyone who saw her that something was wrong. When people asked what was wrong, Amanda's response was, "I haven't been feeling 100 percent." If you pressed about what she had, the answer was always "I don't believe in labels." She would never respond to the question and she refused to face her disease head on – even to herself.

Amanda thought denial would make her condition go away. However, her denial was sending mixed emotional messages to her body, which created stress and further compromised her immune system. All this made her recovery take even longer.

It is impossible to get where you are going if you don't know where you have been. Being honest with yourself is part of the beginning exercise.

When I was stricken with rheumatoid arthritis, I can remember my reaction to the diagnosis. I heard it; I understood it and I even wallowed in self-pity for a brief time. I learned enough about the disease to get an idea how it worked but then let my interest in the details of my disease wane as I shifted my focus to something more positive: getting better. My concern became the process of getting well and how it felt when I was 100 percent. I rejoiced each time I had a pain-free day. I was grateful for every bit of improvement and I relished in flexibility when it appeared.

The goal, once again, for you will be to stay focused on wellness instead of illness. Once you know where you are headed it really doesn't matter how you get there or when. Leave the details and the timeline to a Higher Power.

Thoughts to Consider

What you focus on expands.

Ask – believe – receive.

Denial of your condition can be
counter productive.

Steps to Take

Make a determined statement to begin this
journey. It should statewhat you intend
to accomplish.

Focus your attention on where you want to
be (wellness)not where you are (illness).
Don't be the LUPUS lady.

See your desired future state (wellness) and
welcome everything that comes to help you
get there.

Once you've asked, release control and
leave the details and timeline to a Higher
Power.

Be Open To Answers That Come

An Exercise In Releasing Judgments

Once you've asked, answers will be delivered. Now, you may not always recognize them when they are presented and you may not like the messages that are sent, but the answers will come, nonetheless. Rest assured, you will be guided in this journey and that is the most comforting part of the entire process. The guidance will determine the sources of your potential healing as well as the timing.

For me, simply watching such a phenomenon unfold was the most remarkable thing that happened in each of my journeys to recovery. How the answers I needed kept appearing. They didn't all come at once, but whenever they came - I seemed to be ready. You have heard the saying "The teacher will come when the student is ready." Well, that proved to be true with me. Once I decided I wanted to be well, I just had to be open to the possibilities and they were presented, one after another.

In the best selling book some years ago, *The Celestine Prophecy*, James Redfield wrote of a mission to find a manuscript in Peru that would reveal nine Insights. Throughout the journey to find this manuscript, the main character was provided support, direction and answers to the problems that blocked his progress along the way. The book was full of coincidences, which weren't coincidences at all.

Your journey to wellness will be no different. Once you know specifically where you are headed, and possess a firm intention, the way will become clear. There will be no coincidences on that journey, either. Everything will unfold in the right time and in the right place.

You might doubt and others around you might doubt. Initially, my husband at the time, seemed a little concerned, but eventually he became my most active supporter. He, in fact, ended up being the messenger for the first amazing bit of help the Universe provided.

Not long after stating my intention to find answers outside of conventional medicine for my rheumatoid arthritis, he came home and told me he had been speaking to an old friend about being worried about me. The friend recommended a nutritionist who had worked with many prominent people in town. Without another thought, I took her name and number and called the next day for an appointment.

Put Aside Judgments

Although it was months before I could get in to see Mrs. Dee Kell, the nutritionist, her assistant gave me my first assignment on the phone prior to the initial visit. I was to record everything I ate and drank every day for three weeks. I was to bring this information with me to our first meeting. I did what I was told, three-weeks prior to the meeting for each day I wrote everything that passed my lips. I could already see some items on that list didn't look too good when reduced to writing but being a dutiful patient, I did what I was told. With my task complete and paper in hand, I showed up to her home for my first appointment.

Being somewhat of a professional snob, I was pretty critical that her home was her office. Mrs. Kell's helper was a very sweet woman but not very efficient and I waited more than 45 minutes to get into see her. I was already judging. I was used to efficient, lavishly decorated medical offices and thought those trappings meant I would be getting the very best of care. My attitude changed the moment I met the woman who would change the rest of my life. Right then, all comparisons stopped cold.

Dee Kell, who had her Masters in Nutrition, was warm, genuine and extremely bright - and made me feel as though I was the only person who had ever been seated across from her desk. She wanted to hear everything about me. She asked good questions. When she looked at my food list, she didn't scold, even though she saw some very obviously unhealthy items listed that I had eaten and drunk. Over the months, she began to educate me about basic nutrition, about my body and about how a body is supposed to work. I saw her every month for a year or so.

On the initial visit, she said something to me that turned out to be the most significant message of all, for my condition. She told me that since rheumatoid arthritis was an immune deficiency disease, we were going to concentrate on getting my immune

47

system healthier. Now, that is getting to the root of the problem and it made perfect sense.

She asked me to list all the medications I took and then explained that the drugs I was taking were doing the work my immune system was intended to do and in some cases, suppressing my immune system's function. She continued to say that it is difficult to get the immune system to work properly if something else is doing what it is supposed to do. When that happens, the immune system just shuts down and lets the drugs do the work. All the time we met, Mrs. Kell never asked me to stop taking any medication but I did it anyway. This was my journey and my decision and seemed logical that if I was to build my body back to normal, I had to remove all the obstacles.

I gradually weaned myself off all drugs not only to give my immune system a chance to function on its own but also so I could begin to read my body's normal reactions to my daily routine. Many of the drugs I was taking were speeding up my metabolism or doing other things that were either stimulating or depressing normal function. Mrs. Kell was my first teacher and during the time we were together, I was determined to become her best pupil.

The second most important thing she told me was that there might be something else interfering with the function of my immune system, because of other symptoms I had described. She deduced it was candida albicans, a yeast overgrowth that can become quite invasive and over time can produce very serious and chronic side effects. In order to rid myself of this nasty little problem there was a dietary process I was asked to follow that wasn't going to be easy. Since I wasn't the most disciplined person in the world, I was hoping maybe the candida would just go away quickly with a pill. Sound familiar? Well, that wasn't the method or the timeframe. Of course, today there is a prescription that helps eliminate this much more quickly than the method I used, but an accompanying diet is still helpful.

The longer it took to eliminate the candida in my system, the longer it was necessary to stay on the diet. I found the process pretty tough and began to rationalize maybe this candida wasn't critical after all. Then, along came the reinforcement I needed - very coincidentally - articles began appearing all around me. I picked up a *RedBook Magazine* and there was a huge article on candida albicans and how serious it is. I heard a radio interview on the same topic a few weeks later. There were TV shows dealing with the subject and over the next few months I must have seen dozens of articles to reinforce my need to continue.

Within the first three weeks on the diet, I began to notice more energy and an improvement in my joint swelling and stiffness. I was headed in the right direction. This was the first positive signal since I was diagnosed that all this was paying off. And, it was perfect timing. The dramatic improvement gave me the faith to continue down the path I had chosen – as difficult as it might be. Other answers were being supplied to me, too. I just had to remember to be open and to forget about being judgmental.

There Isn't One Source For All Answers

While I was seeing Mrs. Kell, other methods of help were also being presented. Mrs. Kell had no problem with that and never discouraged my experimentation. Not too long into our

49

relationship, maybe a couple of years, she retired and moved away. She has since passed on.

Her departure was my first lesson not to become totally dependent upon one person or one source. She was a teacher for me, one of many. But because this was my path and my journey, I found that many more messengers were going to be presented to me - some in the form of teachers and some just conveying bits of information. Although Mrs. Kell had gone, I retained the important things she taught me and moved on to find other answers to help. By this time, I was dramatically better in my eyes - even though I was only about 40 percent improved.

Over the next year or so, I began to become more and more aware of the strange places answers popped up. I didn't seek them out necessarily they just started appearing in my life. They will for you, too. You may hear two people discussing an alternative therapy you've always been curious about. That same subject might also show up again in a magazine article at your dentist's office. You might hear about it one more time when a friend calls to tell you about a new book she thinks you should read. When you buy the book, you will find it interesting and want to, at least, try what it says. The Universe is persistent, though, so if you are supposed to try something and don't accept the suggestion the first time, you will probably be reminded again. Forget analyzing the source or even its potential for success, forget all your judgments and just do it. Otherwise that idea will keep gnawing and gnawing at you until you give in.

One example of another important encounter came, when I found myself in the back room of a health food store with a girl named Sunday and a very strange machine. Over and over again, I had to put aside my judgment and trusted in what was being put before me. Sunday, and her Radionics machine ended up being extremely helpful to me over a period of years even though both seemed a little spooky at first. Sunday was a beautiful woman with a little girl voice and absolutely no initial credibility - but she had a gift. She treated me on the machine and taught me about different vitamins and minerals.

The machine was a diagnostic and treatment tool and something I used to help pull toxins out of my body and to treat various conditions by dialing in a variety of frequencies. Of course, the machine would be viewed by anyone else as pure quackery, but it helped me when I was loaded with uric acid or when my body was overly inflamed. It operated on low grade radio frequencies and we'd key-in specific frequencies for various organs, conditions or nutrients. We'd watch a reading that would indicate how healthy I was regarding each.

I felt a little better when I read in *People* magazine that Prince Charles and the Royal Family were into holistic medicine, took homeopathic remedies and were devotees of a number of other alternative processes. A Radionics machine was mentioned for diagnosing illness and diseases in their horses (they probably used it on *themselves*, too, but were too embarrassed to mention it in the article). Now, as strange as it sounds I used that machine for many things and still do today. It helps to reduce radiation after flying, to boost the function of various organs, to de-stress, to control candida and to detox, besides hundreds of other functions. It helped me dramatically. That was one of the therapies I didn't tell anyone else about, except my husband, because my normal friends would have thought I was nuts.

I had dropped all judgment by this time and regardless how it looked, I used anything I could get my hands on to give myself relief since I was going cold turkey with the pain and needed all the help I could find. If the treatment didn't interfere with my immune system, I was willing to try it. Drugs were totally out of the question - even aspirin. So, I found relief with remedies like shark cartilage, evening of primrose oil, liquid calcium, ice packs and ace bandages at night, meditation and my silly machine.

There were other odd remedies that I ran across, which I tried but if I found they didn't work very well for me, I wouldn't continue. The ones that worked, in some way or another, I kept around for a while, at least, as long as I needed them. I was taking natural products to help my symptoms while I did everything I knew how to do to allow my immune system to heal.

For me this was really a trial and error process. There was no formula for finally reaching wellness for me and there won't be a one-size-fits-all formula for you, either. Since no two people are exactly the same and everyone's bodies behave differently, we need a custom approach to facilitate healing.

My remarkable healing journey continued to reveal new modalities with which to experiment. As I moved forward, I learned to value chiropractic for keeping my body comfortable and in alignment, so it could function at peak form. By a process of elimination, I also began a food sensitivity exercise to determine if I was putting stress on my body through things I ingested - foods that I didn't tolerate well. Those intolerances ended up being critical to my healing. I learned I was gluten sensitive and very intolerant of sulfites and nitrates. When I eliminated these three - I, again, had a dramatic improvement. Also, when they were added back, within 36 hours, I had an attack. I also taught myself to meditate and did lots of visualization. I learned about the power of emotions, about affirmations and as this journey unfolded so did my spiritual growth.

Throughout my judgment-free adventure, I did a number of other things that might have seemed radical and extreme but, it wasn't from a sense of desperation, it was from a sense of curiosity. I stumbled on a Reiki practitioner, who aligned chakras. She gave me advice from entities she channeled, about additional vitamins I needed. At first I resisted her advice since I hadn't asked in the first place. The way the message was delivered, I had no way of knowing if she simply made the advice up herself. But, when I resisted, over the course of the next few days, her advice haunted me over and over again until I finally succumbed. I reluctantly took the vitamins and guess what? They helped. So much for, once again, being judgmental.

Much later, I was also drawn to rocks and minerals and learned about the healing properties they held. I would put select stones by my bedside at night. I met a healer, whose talent included both structural and energy work. He helped some. And, I found essential oils interesting and every once in a while used them successfully. I also learned about the benefit of colonics and the use of castor oil packs, an old Edgar Casey remedy for detoxing the liver.

The emotional and spiritual side of my healing got a boost through the support I found with other women, like me, searching for a sense of connectedness. Throughout this time, I built friendships that I never had time for before and found new opportunities for growing my spiritual side, expressing love and having fun.

All this sounds like a lot, but most of it happened over a period of years. Each was of some benefit – but generally the use of these remedies was sporadic instead of routine. I kept trying because I wasn't 100 percent yet. I experienced one or two methods at a time as different messages and messengers appeared. It was wonderful learning about what my body liked and responded to and what it didn't.

Honor The Coincidences

As my journey continued, I began to treat my body with more respect. I welcomed all the information that came to help; books, tapes and new acquaintances. I was open and I saw small amounts of progress with each step I took. There were no coincidences in my life; everything was happening for a reason.

I mentioned earlier about the power of coincidence in referring to one of the reoccurring themes in the *Celestine Prophecy*. To many people, the tone of that book might be too New Age or metaphysical to accept as credible. So, to help balance that reference, I wanted to reinforce my lesson about coincidences in a totally different context.

I was at the wedding of a long time friend, a devout Christian woman, who had just found the man of her dreams at age 50 after being single all her life. While seated in the chapel, I read the program, which chronicled coincidences which had happened in the lives of the bride and groom and had given them so much in common, they were eventually brought together as a couple. At the bottom of the page, after reading fifteen to twenty remarkable events that had occurred in their separate but uniquely linked lives, there was one simple statement in quotes:

"Coincidence is God's way of remaining anonymous."

Accepting a coincidence as providence takes faith. Having faith doesn't need to be born out of a connection to a formal religion. It can come from a sense or an instinct that things will work out for the best. It can be a trusting, perhaps of yourself, perhaps of a higher power. But, overall it requires optimism, and hope.

The process of finding the answers is the most exciting part of this journey. For at every turn doors will be opened to you and marvelous opportunities will present themselves. Some may be methods you've never heard of, some may be the obvious and still others could be modalities that will take every bit of effort to keep from reacting with an, "Are you kidding?" They all will be sent for a reason and in the end - you will find overall healing that is everything you wanted. Just remember, your answers will come in three separate areas; those that help your body, those that help your mind and those that help your spirit.

Each time an answer is delivered to you, consider it. If it feels right, do it. If you are curious, try it. If you are drawn to it and don't know why - jump ahead. Remember the answers that come to you are not a coincidence. They are Divinely inspired.

Thoughts to consider.

Your guidance will determine the sources for
your treatment as well as the timing.

The teachers will come when the student
is ready.

Coincidence is God's way of
remaining anonymous.

The journey to wellness is one we go on
alone. It is an exercise in trusting our
inner voice.

There isn't one source for all answers.

Be patient with your progress. It took time for
your body to breakdown and it will take time
for it to rebuild itself.

Steps to take.

Keep open to the messages and messengers
which appear.

Forget being judgmental. It is
counter-productive.

Start to recognize your feelings.
They will be more important to you than
your intellect during this journey

.

Be Open To Answers That Come From Within
My Body Made Me Do It

W hen answers come to you most are unsolicited and generally a surprise. The process, therefore, needs no formal
planning. It is an exercise in trust. If you believe, as I did, that my
journey was somehow, Divinely led, trust becomes easier.

My journey to wellness was also not an intellectual one. As a
matter of fact, intellect seemed to get in the way, especially if one
begins judging, second-guessing or rationalizing. Wellness is an
exercise in feeling, in trust, and in faith. I just tried to remember I
was embarking on an adventure. I had the big picture of where I
wanted to end up and yet I was leaving all the details to the Universe. I had no idea how I was going to get well. The joy for me
came in watching the path unfold. As it was for me, this experience will be an adventure for you, too.

Your Body The Messenger

In order to be able to experience the true potential of our bodies, we must learn how that marvelous tool communicates with us. One of the methods is the language of feelings. We experience those feelings time and time again on a daily basis, yet most of us simply overlook those signals while we were rushing through life. Because some of us stuff and store our feelings, don't recognize them or ignore them completely - the significance or relevance of these messages are often lost.

In a healing journey – how you feel about something will make a big difference in your selection process. How you feel after you experiment with a new remedy or treatment - it helps a little, a lot or not at all. Again, this is not an intellectual exercise so what you think about it is not nearly as important as how it feels to you.

We are able to pay the most attention to the feelings our body is sending when there is no intellectual or physical interference. That is all too rare because physically, when we take in a host of chemicals daily like caffeine, nicotine and alcohol it dulls or masks our reactions and our true feelings. Stronger drugs such as tranquilizers, pain-killers, anti-depressants and sleeping pills really interfere with getting in touch with the messages our body is sending. Even though some of the stronger feelings manage to squeak through, the whispers get lost. If we could rid our systems of the chemicals that mask our reactions, it would be much easier to understand what our body needs or is trying to tell us.

Most of our feelings take place in the center of our bodies. That is why we have been told to trust our "gut feelings" or "gut instincts". Not only do the gut and brain have common chemical elements but the configuration of those two regions of the body is so similar. Some eastern cultures believe that the messages being sent from the lower center of the body (small and large intestines) are even *more* important to us that what is consciously thought within our brain.

Those feelings are meant to help us, to direct us and to lead us to an easier, healthier life. Let's start with the *gnawing feeling* you get in the pit of your stomach, which *eats* at you to do something. And, eat is the operable word. It's most frequently your body telling you when you're hungry. So, when you do what you're supposed to do - put food in your stomach - the uncomfortable feeling disappears. This is simply a signal to encourage nourishment.

What about the *knot in your stomach*? That usually reminds you something around you is making you very uncomfortable. Maybe it's someone's behavior, something you're seeing or something you've heard that is unpleasant to you. It is a signal that whatever it is - it is creating unhealthy reactions in your body. You should move away from the irritant by turning the channel, hanging up the phone or leaving the room.

There is also the *anxious feeling* we all get when we're rushed or nervous about an upcoming event. You know, the panicky feeling that can occur when you have too much to do and too little time or about to take on something with very little self-confidence. If it's the stressed feeling, it is a signal you are overloaded or trying to do too much. It could mean you should slow down or could mean you are still not totally prepared. If it is the anxious feeling, in general, it could mean you are worrying and in your head instead of being centered, grounded and in the present moment. Take a few, deep slow breaths to get centered and to regain your focus.

When we begin to go over the limit, to push too hard, to do too much or to forget to do what our body needs, it will speak up. Our bodies do not want to feel uncomfortable. Life should flow at a nice even, effortless and worry-free pace. That is possible, and when it occurs, it is heaven. That is also the perfect place to be for healing to occur.

Another feeling is the one that urges us to *run away* from something. It is a physical panicky feeling that is sometimes accompanied by a feeling like your *chest is closing up*. This is a particular feeling I get when I am exposed to toxic smells I cannot tolerate, like some perfumes. It also happens to me with cigarette smoke and bug spray, too.

If your body is like mine, it doesn't like to be around those situations so if I'm in an elevator with a woman wearing heavy perfume, by the time we've reached the next floor, I have pushed my way up to the front, pressed the next button holding my breath and in a panic, rushed out of that door as quickly as possible - regardless of what floor I ended up on. My body moves me out of smelling range at lightning speed. That is a signal for me of contamination - of being around something that is too toxic to my body. There is no benefit in toughing it out; it's time to physically move out of range.

Heart-ache is another beauty. The sad, sad feeling that actually aches in the left side of your chest. It feels like a bottomless pit of emotional hurt that emanates from the center of your being. It is clearly a signal to do something to facilitate relief. It is amazing how your body will tell you when there are even emotional issues that need to be released or resolved so they don't do damage later. So, this is a signal to release them; to do something to get rid of that feeling. It could be crying. Maybe you should call the person you love or miss, and express your feelings from the heart. Perhaps it is simply easier to write a letter that may never be mailed. Maybe it is just talking things out with a friend. Whatever makes your body feel better is the appropriate action to take.

There is also *anxious anticipation*. There is a difference between a stressful, worry and a strong anticipation. Anticipation could foretell something, which could end up being wonderful. It's a little stress and a little excitement all wrapped up into one. When this feeling hits, don't let it paralyze you. That is a *good* signal and should encourage you to forge ahead. Whatever it is will be beneficial to your growth.

Once you begin to focus on your body and learn to recognize the feelings - both good and bad - you will learn the signals your body uses to communicate with you. They are there for a reason. They have always been there, but as we have grown into adulthood, we think we are smarter than our bodies and our brain begins to take over. If you notice, children recognize those signals and express them naturally. They jump up and down when they see something that makes them happy. They push things away they don't like. They are spontaneous, they are real, and they are alive. It is often parents, corporate protocols or political disciplines that encourage us to suppress our feelings; sometimes to mask them totally for such a long period of time that we lose touch with them altogether.

I'm not advocating we always need to speak-up about what we feel to other people, but we must at least be aware of what those feelings are and what they mean to us. The good feeling you get, for example, when something is really right, the proposal, the poem, the painting. Maybe you get goose bumps, get chills or you well up with tears. But, when that special feeling of yours hits, you know whatever it is, is perfect.

Conversely, when things aren't right, when you hear something you know is wrong or someone is telling you a lie, what signals does your body give? Do your eyes dart to another person in the room for confirmation or support? Do you freeze for a split second almost stunned in silence? Do you furrow your brow? Do you look away? To each of us the reaction can be quite different, but it is important to begin to notice the things that are unpleasant in our lives, so that we can start to see patterns, which might require change or some other remedy.

The first time I can remember consciously listening to my body was the methotrexate experience with my rheumatologist. When he suggested it I froze momentarily, I didn't want to say yes or no for a minute, I just looked at him. My second reaction was to pull back, to pull away. I didn't think at that moment, I felt. That is when I told him I needed some time, left and began my journey.

I continued to follow the feelings my body sent as I've made my healing journeys from rheumatoid arthritis, leukemia and countless other incurable conditions to wellness through the following months and years. Through those journeys, I added regimens or remedies that felt right or made me feel better and eliminated those that didn't. My body became my advisor.

Your Body's Signals

Throughout my adult life, I had been receiving signals from my body about my health but, like most of you, I ignored them. I didn't even realize my body was trying to communicate with me. When my eyes would begin to feel heavy at 6:30 at night because I was so exhausted, I'd just drink some caffeine or smoke cigarettes and continue to forge ahead. When I was anxious and overstressed, I sedated myself with alcohol to calm down and relax; instead of releasing the stress, I masked it. I pushed and pushed and pushed for years ignoring anything that had to do with my body, and me. I always put myself last. And, finally, my body gave me a major wake-up call. Attacks of excruciating pain in various joints, in the middle of the night, that eventually developed into rheumatoid arthritis. Because I wasn't listening to the whispers, my body had to yell.

If you experience continual feelings of discomfort in your body, it could be a pattern to which you need to pay attention. The goal is to get rid of discomfort when it happens. Your body is trying to help. It wants to feel perfect, that's why it tells us exactly what it needs and when it needs it. This process is the opposite of being driven by habit, which is the way most of us operate. Our body not only guides us in healthy choices in a physical sense but in healthy choices in relationships, too. Everything we do and feel affects our health, which is why feelings are so important to begin to understand.

Our feelings are one of the ways our spirit speaks to us - in order to give us guidance in our lives. Feelings are the language of the soul.

Your Body's Other Signals

In your journey to wellness, you are given lots of choices and lots of opportunities to become healthy. The way to know if you are making the right choices is by paying attention to the reaction of your body. Your body will send obvious signals to you when something is either good or bad.

On more than one occasion, my body actually walked me into a place I never would have considered going. You know, "the devil made me do it" compulsion. Once, I was *drawn* into a health food store. It was one of those old, cluttered and dusty ones, not the kind of environment in which I would ever enjoy browsing but I automatically walked in. That is where I met another contact who became a wonderful teacher who helped me explore the value of specific vitamins, minerals and other nutrients.

Unrelated to healing, but another perfect example of how we are often drawn, without conscious thought, to a place we needed to go. This situation involved my former husband, Steve. One afternoon, Steve was headed down the freeway to come home and was in sort of a 'zone' while driving. I always kidded him about being a Pisces and being prone to "zones" anyway - but during this instance, his car was being pulled off at an earlier exit called Indian School Road (four exits ahead of our normal turn-off to come home). He caught himself as the car began turning onto the off ramp. He whipped the car back to the left, nearly hitting another car, yet managing to keep control and to head in what he considered to be the right direction. Before he got to the normal exit to go home, his cell phone rang and it was a client who had papers ready for him to sign. The client's office was east, just off the Indian School Road exit.

The things our bodies know are amazing. And, they are so eager to help. Another signal we are given is a *reaction*. You know, when your head turns involuntarily and you catch sight of something perhaps you connect as important, perhaps not. This is precisely what happened to me just the other day when preparing to leave for a meeting. I had finished getting dressed and was walking through the master bedroom. My head turned, for no apparent reason, and I noticed a folder on my bed that was important to take with me that day. Had I not been directed to look in that direction, I would have missed the folder I needed for the meeting or would have had to go back into the bedroom to get it before I left the house.

I will also share another bit of body wisdom. A good friend and past-business associate of mine, named Shirley, had just flown in from Denver that day and stopped by my house as we had arranged. It was about 5:00 PM and we were going to run down the street and grab a quick bite to eat before calling a client of ours in Australia with a 15-hour time difference. The call was to occur at 7:00 PM, M.S.T. It was important to reach him at the start of his business day. While we were standing in the kitchen, Shirley's arm rose slightly and she unconsciously looked at her watch and said, "Oh, it's 5:45 PM, we still have plenty of time for dinner and to call at 7:00 PM, lets go." She had not intentionally checked her watch because she knew we had plenty of time, but when her arm rose, she commented on the time and off we went.

We returned home from dinner in plenty of time and made the call promptly at 7:00 PM - we found we were an hour too late

- the client had already left for a meeting. Shirley had forgotten to re-set her watch from Denver time when she arrived in Phoenix. We should have made the call at 6:00 PM, Denver time. A nice reminder her body gave her at 5:45 PM, but neither one of us got the message.

These things happen to us all the time, and when we begin to notice, it becomes truly entertaining. Our bodies remind us to do things, to make life flow easier and simpler. We're just usually too busy or moving too fast to pay much attention. Learning to trust our bodies and to listen to their wisdom makes the healing journey proceed much quicker and life in general, flow a whole lot easier.

Spontaneous thought is another way in which our bodies facilitate communication for us. Spontaneous thought is when things pop into our heads uninvited. Now, it is much easier to receive such information if your mind is uncluttered from the day - a perfect reason to learn meditation. When our minds are uncluttered, such thoughts are easier to recognize. Only then can we hear the subtle messages - before the yells are needed.

When random thoughts pop into my mind they are usually important. Sometimes they are answers to questions I have posed about one thing or another. For example: a great gift idea I had been concerned about, surfaces when least expected - but always in time. I don't have to consciously say, "Now what should I get him?", yet my mind answers back. The answer or idea comes, when it's ready. This is real spontaneous stuff and generally out of context. I could be in the shower and there's a flash reminder that I still have clothes in the dryer. A clear mind can help you receive those wonderfully practical messages and the ones that will help guide you to better health.

Dreams are still another way our bodies communicate - they are part of that built-in, inner guidance system, too. Dreams and I back then never connected but I know others who found answers to their problems quite frequently through dreams and today I do, too. Some of us keep a pad and pencil by our bed and record dreams. There are even people around who do dream interpretation, to help novices, like me.

One of the most obvious ways our bodies facilitate communication is with kinesiology, a method of muscle testing many chiropractors use to ask our bodies for information. Kinesiology also can be used in other ways to access information from our subconscious or Higher Self. Some believe the information comes from some unknown information source in the body (perhaps cells); others believe it is the subconscious and still others believe it is universal knowledge we are able to tap into during the process. For me, kinesiology was one of the first and most dramatic illustrations of body talk.

Regardless of how your body chooses to communicate with you, you will find methods that are the easiest to grasp coming to you first, and others following later.

Christiane Northrup M.D., I mentioned earlier as a nationally recognized holistic expert in women's health, believes that listening to your body is one of the five immediate steps you can take to heal yourself. "That means tuning-in and taking care of yourself. Start by resting when you're tired. And eating when you're hungry. And saying no when you've reached your limits. The more you honor these internal messages, the more inner guidance will come your way. As your powers of intuition develop, you'll soon know what your body wants and needs. It's uncanny - but 100 percent reliable."[9]

Thoughts to consider.

This journey is an exercise in trust. It is Divinely led.

Your body is also a messenger.

Kinesiology is a wonderful way for your body to communicate some providers use it in their practice.

Steps to take.

Start listening to your feelings – they are the language of your soul.

Be aware when your body makes you do something like turn your head, look at your watch or your eyes keep drifting to something. Do it.

Learn which signals your body sends when you are upset or when you are really happy.

Be aware of spontaneous thoughts – when things pop into your mind or if a thought haunts you over and over. Act on them.

Write down vivid dreams and see if they speak to you.

---

[9] Christiane Northrup, M.D., "*How to Choose a Health Miracle In Your Life,*" From a promotional flier, 1999, 5.

Forget intellect as it relates to judging,
second-guessing or rationalizing – it will get
in the way.

Take Action Without Fear

You Can't Move Ahead
If You Don't Move At All

T he secret to getting ahead is getting started. This is not a profound quote from a wise old sage, it came from the inside of a fortune cookie and it's completely true. To be successful you must begin with the first step. No fairy-godmother with a magic wand will make this happen for you; you will need to physically get out of your chair or off your couch and do it yourself. I guess this chapter could be summed up with the classic quote: "God helps those who help themselves."

Also, for those of you content to let a Higher Power deliver your miracle, I am here to provide a reality check. Although there is certainly a spiritual component to any healing journey, every individual still has to also do his or her part to make it work. As most everyone knows, prayer can play a significant role in facilitating wellness but in the end, it is up to us to act on that which is given. The Universe, God, Spirit, your Higher Self, whatever you choose to call it - answers prayers in ways we might not understand or even recognize, but prayers are always answered in one way or another. The key is to ask for the right thing and then be willing to step up to the plate and try what is presented. Let me share a story, with which you might be familiar, that illustrates this point perfectly.

A man was sitting on the roof of his house during a raging flood. He prayed and prayed for God to save him from the rising waters. In the course of those prayers a young boy floated by while holding on to a large log, "Jump on," said the boy. "There's plenty of room."

"No, that doesn't look too sturdy. I'll just wait here, God will deliver me," replied the man as he kept on praying. Soon, the water reached the second story window. By that time a group of people came by in a rowboat. They yelled, "There isn't much room inside, but you can hang on to the side - jump and we'll pull you with us."

"No, the man said, that seems pretty risky. I'm praying to God to help me." The water continued to rise and this time it was nearly to his chest. Soon, deep in prayer, the man heard a helicopter hovering overhead and saw a rope dangling from the open door.

"Grab on to the rope, we'll pull you up." They yelled at him from the chopper.

"I don't think I'm strong enough to do that," the man yelled back. "Something else will come along - I'm in God's hands."

The water continued to rise and finally the man became submerged and drowned. When he reached heaven and came face to face with his Maker, the man impeached, "Why didn't you answer my prayers? Why did you abandon me, God?"

"Abandon you?" God replied, "I sent you a log, a boat and then a helicopter."

This is a beautiful lesson to show us how answers may come we don't understand and why we should not judge. It also teaches us that prayer alone is not enough without some personal action. Yes, you are also responsible for what you do with what is given.

Adopt that Nike slogan that said, "Just do it." Even if you're wrong, you may learn something valuable in the process. I found every single thing I did taught me something either about releasing judgment, learning more about the other components of healing or about faith. The key is to act.

If you are an action person, this part will be easy. If you are a person who thinks, plans, prays and strategizes but is not very action oriented, then you have to find something to motivate you. Just becoming well isn't always enough motivation for some people. So, dig deep and ask yourself, "What is the real reason I want to get well?"

It could be relationships with others that will propel you into action - like a new significant other, an adorable grandchild, a new friend or a pet. All of a sudden being ill or not being in the picture makes a difference. Or, it could be an interest outside yourself that will stimulate you to move: a new hobby, a new job, even discovering a new author who has an inventory of books you'd love to wade through. It may also be simply a fear of dying and you want time to get your spiritual act together; that is fine, too. Or, it can be because you just *want* to.

The sluggish sort of individual who is not prone to jumping into projects will certainly need to identify the motivation that will thrust him or her into tackling this journey. And even for that person, it may take some gusto, enthusiasm and energy but it is certainly possible.

Do Many Others Use Alternative Medicine?

Well, you'll be one of millions. Consumers are getting smarter. That's why over ten years ago, in 1997, Americans made 627 million visits to practitioners of alternative medicine and spent $27 billion of their own money (not covered by insurance) to pay for alternative therapies. In contrast, Americans made only 386 million visits to their family doctor. Harvard Medical School estimates that one out of every two persons in the United States between the ages of 35 and 49 used at least one alternative therapy during 1997. That is a growth of 47.3 percent since 1990.[10] That study concludes that people using alternative medicine are certainly not ignorant. They are predominately well-educated, affluent baby boomers.

In 2000, it was estimated that 71 percent of adults over the age of 50 now use some kind of alternative medicine such as acupuncture and herbal medicine. The same study found that 62 percent of adults of all ages used those modalities.[11]

As more people venture out to try alternative treatments, they find for the most part these alternatives are harmless. No side effects and nothing to damage one's body. There are a few exceptions but even when they do damage they don't kill us. I searched

---

[10] Eisenberg, David M., et al, "Trends In Alternative Medicine Use In The United States," 1990-1997. *Journal of the American Medical Association*, 280: November 11 (1998),1569-75.
[11] National Institute on Aging , 2002. *Survey of 848 respondents:* University of Michigan. (Washington, DC: National Institute on Aging , 2002).

and searched to find statistics about the mortality rate from alternative treatments and couldn't find any - unlike what I found for allopathic care.

Isn't Alternative Medicine Full Of Quacks?

As enlightened as I believe people are today, I still run into individuals who say alternative medicine is weird and really doesn't work. There may be many reasons for this, among them appearance. Many practitioners aren't getting rich by doing the good work they do - and simply don't *look* successful. Their offices are less than modest or in a low rent district. Their office furniture is second hand or inexpensive. Their office staff is minimal, if they have any staff at all.

The truth is, when a practitioner spends much more time with a patient, as naturopaths and holistic physicians do and they don't have the benefit of large surgical fees, for example, they simply earn less money. Add to that the fact that these practitioners probably charge less than a normal doctor visit because quite often, what they do isn't covered by insurance. We are conditioned to believe that an impressive office and flashy accoutrements equate to skill and knowledge. That is not the case and certainly not the case with these folks most of whom are dedicated professionals - many who possess extraordinary healing gifts.

If you are still concerned, ask questions - just as you should of your medical professionals. It is apparent that not every physician finished at the top of his or her class - so when you look at the odds - 33 percent of all medical physicians had to fall in the bottom third. Therefore, I do the same thing in selecting alternative providers that I do in selecting medical practitioners, I ask questions. I ask how long they have been practicing. I also use the referral method and occasionally, I'll check with the State Medical Board or other governing body to monitor complaints. For referrals I ask someone I trust - like another provider in the field - who is good in a particular specialty. Peer or patient referrals are best. If you can't find any, pick up publications from the industry and look for articles about or written by various professionals. Sometimes with alternative practitioners, I will look at their ads and then call and ask a few questions. If I am drawn to them, I call. The one thing that is different about alternative providers is that some have few if any credentials but have incredible natural gifts for healing. You can spot them a mile away and they are the ones I find generally come to me from referrals from others - or through coincidence, which I always honor. You'll see why later.

It is important to check on anyone who treats you; although someone who is incompetent in alternative medicine will only waste your time and money whereas an incompetent in the medical field could potentially do much more damage.

Finally, don't assume someone is a "quack" just because his or her methodology sounds unusual. I have had some pretty strange things done to me and they have all worked. Ear "coning" for example is a terrific way to remove wax from one's ears. They don't use whatever method a typical E.N.T. specialist does today; they gently insert a paper cone and light it on fire. Well, the paper doesn't burst into flames or anything like that - the material burns very, very slowly and the trapped smoke and heat draws the wax out into the paper. It is amazingly effective and a very relaxing process. So, to me - a little "quackery" can be surprisingly helpful and fun.

I just caution people to not let their intellect get in the way and second-guess their way out of the alternative area. Just because it is something you don't initially understand - doesn't mean it won't be good for you and won't work. A little bit of skepticism is no reason for inaction.

Remember, Conventional Medicine Is Not Traditional Medicine

As you move forward with alternative medicine, remember its roots. That may get you more excited about venturing out. Although most people continue to refer to conventional medicine as traditional medicine and everything else outside of that realm as alternative, that is not correct. Traditional means based on or related to tradition. Modern medicine, as we know it, only truly began in the 20th century. Acupuncture, Auverdic Medicine, Chiropractic, Nutritional Therapy, Sound Therapy, Yoga, Massage, Hydrotherapy, Imagery and Visualization, Essential Oils and other forms of alternative medicine go back thousands of years. I spent a long time researching each of these modalities through a variety of sources and cross checking the information in several books that mention of the options available. I knew most were extremely old but really had no idea now far back many of the methods originated.

Ayurvedic Medicine, for example, began with the sages of ancient India 5,000 years ago. Acupuncture was developed in

China thousands of years ago and both these modalities are still used in their countries of origin as well as all over the world. Massage, which many people consider a feel-good treatment and not a credible method for healing is actually the most natural of natural remedies. Most forms have been around for at least 5,000 years. Nutritional therapy, also acknowledged for its benefits but not necessarily given the credit it deserves as a highly effective healing modality, dates as far back as Hippocrates, who said in 400 B.C., "Let food be your medicine and medicine be your food." Chiropractic, although started formally in 1895, was originally invented by the ancient Greeks in 1250 B.C. It was the Greeks who first considered treating muscular and skeletal disorders through manipulation of the spine.

One of the more unusual forms, Hydrotherapy, was first used by Hippocrates in the fourth century B.C. and has been part of the healing tradition of nearly every civilization from ancient Greece and Egypt to Rome, where virtually all medicine was practiced at the public baths. Imagery and Visualization have been considered healing tools in practically all of the world's cultures including Western Indian tribes such as Navajos as well as the Ancient Egyptians and Greeks such as Aristotle and Hippocrates. Sound therapy appeared about 2,500 years ago when the Greek mathematician and philosopher, Pythagoras, developed 'prescriptions' of music to help his students work, relax, sleep and wake up better. Today it is used to regulate heart beat and ease pain, as well as to relax. Essential Oils and their use topically, diffused or through aromatherapy can be documented in ancient Egyptian hieroglyphics and Chinese and Eastern Indian manuscripts as well as references in the Bible.

The longevity of these methods cannot be questioned and the reason they have lasted all this time is because they work. Now, doesn't hearing a little about their history make the thought of exploring some of those options more intriguing?

So, specifically what is the action are we supposed to take, when are we supposed to take it and what if we make a mistake? Let's start with the last question first and it will answer all three. The most interesting part of the healing journey process is that there are no mistakes. The process is cumulative and progressive and perfect. Everything will come in perfect order. It is your job to have faith and to follow. You will not find one guru, one doctor, or one adviser to tell you what to do and explain it all to you. The process does not work that way. There isn't a silver bullet, a quick fix or a one-source method for answers, either. It may not even make sense at the time. You have to believe that whatever is presented to you is something you are supposed to try. In the process of trying you will learn information beneficial to your healing. One source might only help you five percent but you will be five percent ahead of where you were. Remember, it is irrelevant how slow you go as long as you are headed in the right direction. Any improvement is good improvement.

Find Measurements To Chart Your Progress

I had dramatically different healing journeys with my two most significant conditions. One condition presented symptoms on which the improvement was easy to gauge. The other did not and the measurement had to be managed another way.

With the rheumatoid arthritis I looked for pain relief, less joint swelling and less stiffness. In other words, total symptomatic improvement. I also watched for improvement in my energy and for a healthy look to return to my skin and hair. My leukemia left me, on the other hand, with a very exhausted feeling but the doctors tracked the severity of my condition through my blood work. I had a high white count and a high lymph count. So to gauge my progress, I looked for more energy and to feel more like my old self but I also wanted my blood work to return to normal.

The monitoring of my white count and lymph count required some doing. The doctor at the University of Arizona Cancer Center was content to see me every three months and chart my progress. That was not enough for me. Since I was taking an active role in the healing process, I found a holistic medical office that would draw my blood monthly, send it to the lab and fax me a copy of the CBC results. That way I could chart the progress of my white blood cell count as well as the progress of my lymph count. Don't be afraid to take the initiative in your own case and to ask for information or make arrangements that work for you.

I wasn't discouraged if my white count and lymph count didn't drop dramatically or as fast as I had hoped each time. I watched every month to make sure the white count, in particular, didn't increase and even if it simply remained stable I figured I was ahead of the game because the doctors expected it to spike up and down routinely. Spiking up was no option for me. The timing for improvement would take as long as it took, so I was patient with the results of each report. I waited with anticipation for the results each month and celebrated to myself when each fax report came. I watched each count drop and drop until finally both reached the normal rage with no spikes upward. It took nearly two years and that was perfectly fine with me.

You will find a way to measure your progress, too. Keep a record via charts and journals and remember, the timeline will not be yours. It will happen when it does. You are only in charge of making sure you're headed in the right direction. Every new experience should help you improve - even a little. Add that knowledge, remedy or information to your wellness regime and build one upon the other. If your experience doesn't seem to help in some way that you can identify - let that one go and simply move on. But, even at that - I'll bet you learn a great lesson from every experience, perhaps releasing judgment or about a modality that will serve you well later.

You Have To Be Willing To Change

Some action might necessitate making changes in your normal routine or your normal way of thinking. Change is good; change is progress. Illness often forces us to look at situations or conditions we have ignored in our lives on many different levels; the important thing is to dig up the courage to tackle them and to be courageous.

There are a number of reasons why people resist change, even if they know change will be good for them. Most every reason is based on fear. "What will my friends think?" "I can't afford it right now." "I'm not ready yet." "I might fail." "People might laugh at me." "I don't know enough, yet." "It might hurt my image." "I don't know if I can trust them." "I might lose my friends." "It's too hard to do." "Who knows how I might end up." "I don't have the energy" "I might hurt someone's feelings." "I don't have any personal support." This fear needs to be replaced by faith.

In creating wellness, you have to let go of excuses and the need for validation. Sometimes you just have to let go of what is not working, like an overly stressful job, old ideas and beliefs or unhealthy relationships. One of the reasons people don't heal is because they are afraid of the pain of letting go. Ask for help in finding the courage to let go if it is necessary and ask for the strength to deal with the change when it comes because sometimes it will be thrust upon you. Those requests would be effective prayers.

In order to heal, leave those parts of your life, which no longer serve you, behind. As you release them, you will make room for new and better experiences and relationships.

A wonderful example comes to mind of a bookkeeper I had employed some time ago. She had been suffering with gout in her big toe. It was very painful and she complained to me about it more than once. After watching her suffer, I offered a suggestion. "Teresa, you might want to quit wheat, shellfish and red meat for a few days. It will help lower your uric acid level and give your body a chance to recover from this." I said. She whipped around and stated defiantly, "Well, I'm not going to change my *whole life*." Hearing her reaction, my sympathy ceased and so did my input. Change and personal responsibility are key to any successful healing.

I adored reading Bernie Siegel, M.D.'s books especially, *Love, Medicine & Miracles*. In that particular book he talks about the three kinds of patients he experienced in his practice. The victims, who give up and die, the 60 to 70 percent in the middle, who do what they're told, but rarely make hard decisions on their own. This group, he recounted, resists making radical changes in their lifestyle and are loaded with excuses as to why they aren't more aggressive about wellness. Finally, there are the exceptional patients who refuse to play the victim to a disease. They educate themselves, they participate in their health care, and they demand dignity and control. They ask questions and are sometimes considered uncooperative or difficult as patients. They aren't afraid to make lifestyle changes and they are the most likely to get well. I would surmise that these patients are probably the first to use complimentary methods to integrate into their conventional care or may select a totally alternative route if they get a doom and gloom prognosis.

The exceptional patients Dr. Siegel identifies are not afraid to take action. They accept risk as a means for ultimate reward.[12]

Releasing The Fear

When we become ill it is a logical reaction to become gripped by fear. At first, we fear what might be wrong. Then when the diagnosis comes, we fear the prognosis. Then we begin to fear the pain or complications that may result from the progression of our condition or from the suggested treatment. Soon we begin to fear death and being taken before we are ready. There are

---

[12] Bernie S. Siegel, M.D., *Love Medicine & Miracles*, (New York: Perennial Library, Harper & Row Publishers, 1998), 24, 26.

lots of places along the way where fear creeps in and grabs us. Don't let fear dictate the actions you take. Once you are committed to wellness, learn to release fear and have faith.

Fear can do terrible things to people's lives. It will make us cling to the familiar, regardless of whether the familiar is really right for us. We might stick with a doctor longer than we should because we're afraid to try someone or something else. It could make us also blindly accept a treatment that is recommended without asking any questions or respecting our own feelings. Haven't you sometimes felt that a recommendation just didn't "feel right" to you, yet you went ahead with it anyway? Letting go of fear means trusting ourselves and our feelings.

The other day I opened the newspaper and was amazed at what I saw. It was the perfect example of a fear-based therapy. The article was announcing a new prophylactic treatment for women genetically prone to breast cancer. It stated that women with a high risk or propensity toward the disease had a new option. The headline read: *Mastectomy May Extend Life For Gene Carriers.* The article went on to state that a recent study was the first to estimate how much time a "mastectomy in advance" would buy for a woman with a sharply increased risk of breast cancer. Of course, this was based on medical studies (scientific studies). Mayo Clinic researchers had said the surgery could reduce the breast cancer risk by 91 percent but they didn't quantify the benefit in added years of life. Some other studies did try to quantify additional years, assuming the woman would actually contract cancer that was incurable. It never ceases to amaze me how fear can motivate some people to do almost anything.

Fear can also keep a person from acting. You have heard of people who have become paralyzed by fear. That may happen to you - with a bad diagnosis and prognosis. It actually did for me - for a couple days after the Leukemia diagnosis, until I decided I could sit there and wallow in self-pity and grow worse and worse or I could do something about it.

If fear is paralyzing you or is causing you to do something you really don't want to do, you might ask a Higher Power for guidance to make the right decisions. Or, you could simply turn it over and let go. Or, have the confidence to trust your body and yourself in the process. Then, nurture and love yourself every day, do what brings you joy and be grateful for the good in your life.

The following includes steps you can take to replace fear-motivated behavior with love-motivated behavior:

> Since there are only two basic emotions - love and fear, the more you can stay in a state of love, the less you will be overcome by fear. Ask for help with that.

> Begin to meditate and first thing every morning - fill yourself with light and love on a daily basis. At some point, there won't be room for fear-based feelings.

> Learn to live in the present moment. Fear is rooted in the past or future. In the past it is magnified by negative, old experiences. If you can replace those destructive feelings with a centered, present mind it will be much more productive. A future focus allows for fear of the unknown. If you insist on projecting ahead in your day-to-day thinking, replace that fear with trust that the perfect result will be delivered. Those adjustments will make it easier to maintain a state of love within.

Stop negative thoughts and negative self-talk. If you can't think or say anything positive about yourself, don't think or say anything at all.

Learn to reframe negative experiences that happened in your past. See these situations as gifts that were given to you to help shape the person you are today. They may have taught you how not to be or made it necessary for you to develop other traits that have benefited you in later years.

Instead of worry, which is fear-based, let go and turn your troubles over to God, some other Higher Power, or something else and then forget them. Some societies use "worry dolls". People give each of the little dolls one of their worries to handle so they no longer have to, then, they forget the issue.

Do more things in your life that make you smile and bring you joy.

Learn to nurture and love yourself more. You can't give to others if you are empty yourself. Take time for the things you love.

Since your healing will be dramatically affected by your attitude and by how well you recognize and deal with your emotions, learning to minimize fear in your life will be very helpful. Of course, perfection is not a realistic goal and all of us experience fear-based emotions from time to time. So, instead of worrying that negative emotions might crop into your life and concentrating on their elimination, why not concentrate on filling your life with more healthy thoughts? This is a good time to learn to focus on the desired outcome instead of the problem that exists.

Reflect On Yourself And Others In Your Life

Holistic healing is an active state not a passive one. In conventional medicine, we can be passive and let the physician assume all responsibility. In the holistic model, we have the primary role. So, it is up to us to become aware, to take action and to make any changes necessary for our success. In the mind-body-spirit model, self-reflection is also a part of the process. There is no reason to be fearful of self-reflection; it is healthy and beneficial. That is most likely the area in holistic healing that strikes the most fear in the hearts of practitioners - emotions - especially old buried emotions.

As I mentioned before, a great tool to begin this process is *You Can Heal Your Life*, by Louise Hay, to reveal the emotional root cause for the particular illness or condition you have. There you might find a clue to unlock more answers that can facilitate part of your wellness. Even the most minor illness often provides a chance to look at yourself and your life in a different way. With my first major illness, when I referred to Louise Hay's book and looked under Rheumatoid Arthritis, I saw something I didn't initially understand, "Deep criticism of authority. Feeling very put upon." I didn't get it at first.

"How could that be?" I said to myself. "I am very respectful of others. I was a good daughter and was dutiful in that role. I certainly didn't act-up or cause problems." After more thought I still had trouble applying this to me, "I respected all of my bosses in the early years and realized my role as an employee. They loved my work and things were most generally positive. I was always a good person."

Then I looked further. The way I ended up was my first clue. I ended up an entrepreneur; I became my own boss. Not out of resentment, I thought, but based on a desire to control my own destiny. I didn't ask for help from others - maybe it was pride or maybe it was ignorance. I trusted myself more and preferred to make my own mistakes. I could see the imperfections in others and thought those imperfections might contribute to less than 'perfect' advice, so I decided I'd rather trust myself. I had found a way to live without much authority in my life - regardless of how premature that jump to entrepreneurship may have been, and how much stress it eventually caused. I'd rather suffer the stress than take orders from others - especially others who might not know what I knew.

I developed a disease that stopped me from continuing with that paradigm. Over the years of my healing journey, I learned to put aside judgments and accept answers to my healing which came from others - even imperfect individuals. I learned to accept answers from unusual sources and help from people I never would have considered my equals. I learned to seek advice and to take it once it was given. I also learned to love myself more and learned to go within for guidance. I became more humble, more spiritual and more contented with wherever life took me. I learned to let go of control and be less attached to the "specific" outcome. In the process my physical self was healing, I was more open to healing emotional issues and grew closer to God. In all instances, I was taking action and making changes.

Others will find their paths much different. A book such as Louise Hay's may not feel right at all, it might be more meaning-ful to begin by redefining your priorities. A redefinition that puts achieving your wellness first and perhaps, one that begins to open you up to the love of yourself and others.

My second major illness, leukemia, carried with it a totally different issue to be addressed. The morning after I heard the news of my potential illness, I went to the desk in my bedroom and picked up Caroline Myss's book *Anatomy of the Spirit*. I opened it to parts I had highlighted when I read through it the first time, years prior. I settled on a very meaningful paragraph that said: "Unquestionably, a strong link exists between physical and emotional stresses and specific illnesses. The connection has been well documented for instance, with regard to heart disease and hypertension and the so-called Type-A personality. My particular and spiritual insights, however, have shown me that emotional stresses or dis-eases are the root causes of all physical illnesses. Moreover, certain emotional and spiritual crises correspond quite specifically to problems in certain parts of the body. For instance, people who come to me with heart disease have had life experiences that led them to block out intimacy and love from their lives. People with low back pain have had persistent financial worries; people with cancer often have unresolved connections with the past, unfinished business and emotional issues; people with blood disorders frequently have deep-seated conflicts with their families of origin."[13]

The last two concepts really resonated with me. What flashed in my mind was an experience I had as a child, one I didn't remember but was later told about. At age five, my mother was

---

[13] Caroline Myss, Ph.D., *Anatomy of the Spirit*, (New York: Three Rivers Press, Harmony Books,1996), 66.

sitting on my bed - as she always did before she said goodnight - telling me stories about her youth or just talking about the old days. As many children do, I asked if I was adopted. The trigger might have been that I was a blonde, blue-eyed tall youngster with parents were dark haired and brown-eyed or it may have just popped into my head. My mother, who thought lying was the worst sin of all, said "Yes you are." My parents had never told me about my adoption, probably because of my mother's fear I would not love her. So, I know she responded only as a reaction to my question. I panicked and this five-year old began talking about the dog, the weather, tomorrow and rattled on and on about other meaningless things. I guess I wanted to keep my Mother from saying anything more. I think she was relieved, perhaps hoping I had not heard her answer. She didn't continue the conversation and didn't say another word about it for many, many years. I have absolutely no memory of this incident, and my adoption was never discussed again. When I was 18 years of age, my mother told me I was adopted and recounted this story.

I don't know how one survives a "black-out" experience such as this without some type of damage later. Well, this must be *it*, I thought. Ironically, this realization gave me some peace by identifying this incident. "Now, there is something I can do to facilitate my healing on an emotional level," I thought. That morning I talked to Steve about the book and what popped into my head. Still depressed about the recent news, a glimmer of light began to appear as I recounted the passage in the book and my revelation about what I considered the root cause - emotionally. I knew I was right. I had found a place to begin. I found the start of my power to heal.

Later that day, I spent some time alone thinking about that incident as a child. I did what Paige Jackson, a very gifted woman who helps individuals on emotional clearing recommends - I re-framed it. I sat cross-legged on my bed and imagined myself back in Kewanee, Illinois in 1949, in my bedroom off the kitchen of our house on Garfield Street. I became the mother sitting on the edge of the bed and talked to the little girl lying there. This time the mother was armed with all the knowledge, wisdom and love available in the Universe. I said all the things my dear mother would not have recognized were necessary to help me through this trauma. I said what my mother wasn't equipped to say.

When that innocent little child asked the adoption question, I responded with a slow, dramatic pause that helped illustrate the magnitude of the question. Once I was asked *the* question, I then said, "Oh, Sandy. You have to be *very special* to be adopted be-cause a child who is adopted is chosen. She is picked-out of *all* the children in the world to be loved and adored by her new moth-er and father."

"But, Momma, aren't I that special?" the child asked plea-dingly. "Let me tell you a story about a *very, very special* little girl who was adopted by parents who think she is the best little girl in the world." And, she proceeded to tell the story of how a woman with a little boy found out she was going to have another child. The little boy was just reaching pre-school age when she and the boy left a bad marriage. She had to work and support both herself and the child. With a new baby coming, what would she do? She could not stay home with the baby because she had to work to support herself and her son. She was confused and upset. Then, she heard about two people who wanted a baby desperately. She agreed to put her baby up for adoption."

"When the baby girl was born, the mother took one look at the child and wanted to keep her. She was beautiful, sweet and a very special child. The biological mother was changing her mind about the adoption. She didn't know how she would manage with two little children, but she would try. Then she met the husband and wife who wanted a baby so badly. When she saw them in the hospital she knew instantly that they would give her baby a wonderful life and a wonderful home. She knew the adoption was the right thing to do. She said the moment she saw them," This is your baby girl - she is beautiful, she is special and now she belongs to you."

The little five-year old lie in bed, her eyes wide open listening to every word and imagining she was every bit as special as this adopted little child. "Momma, am I that special? Am I as special as that little adopted girl?" she asked with hope and anticipation.

"You *are* that little girl, sweetheart." her mother said. And they both hugged with joy. The little girl felt treasured and reassured and the mother knew she had told the truth and was truly loved, too. It was the perfect ending.

I sat and cried knowing how happy and secure the little girl felt and how happy and secure I was with the new way this event turned out. A flood of contentment swept over me and I felt peace for the first time about this quite unfinished piece of business in my life. I had begun to take action right away to begin the process of healing.

But, sometimes there is more than one answer to a question. I wasn't content that I had explored every emotional avenue - so I picked up Louise Hay's book, as well. She said the root cause of leukemia was something slightly different, but something to consider nonetheless. I pursued that path, as I covered earlier in an earlier chapter and realize for me there were two elements emotionally for me that needed fixing - the unfinished business with my family of origin and finding joy once again. The second part wasn't able to be fully accomplished until seven months later. So you see, with alternative methods it doesn't matter if something is precisely the correct remedy or if it happens when you think it should. Everything you do will be perfect at the time. That single emotional issue was something that clearly needed to be cleaned-up in my life and whether the root cause was unfinished family business or finding joy - I could benefit from both.

There are other ways to begin claiming your power to heal on the emotional (mental) level. You can begin by actively loving yourself more. In that regard, try to do more things that make you happy. If you loved fishing but never took the time, a fishing trip might be the first vacation you plan. If you love to play cards but never had the time, you might join a bridge or poker club. If it is just seeing your children more often or reading a good book - you should begin to fit that into your schedule. Action is the operative word, here. Intentions are great and a good first step, but only thinking about the things you can do, won't work - you must act.

Life is too short and unpredictable to ignore experiences that truly bring you joy. And, the end result is that by experiencing that joy, you are strengthening your immune system and nurturing your self-giving and self-loving tendencies.

Thoughts to consider.

God helps those who help themselves.

There are no mistakes on a healing journey.
You will learn something from
every experience.

There is no silver bullet.

The healing process is cumulative,
progressive and perfect.

Any improvement is good improvement.

Leave behind the parts of your life that no
longer serve you.

Every emotion is either love or fear – let go
of fear.

We have control over the emotions
we choose.

By filling our lives with more love, it leaves
less room for fear.

Holistic healing is an active state not a
passive one.

Steps to take.

The secret to getting ahead is getting started.

Identify the reason you want to get well so
you have a real motive stored in
your subconscious.

Find measurements to chart your progress.
That way you can keep track of how well
you are doing.

Embrace change - change is good and
change is progress.

Replace fear-motivated behavior with love-motivated behavior (use the list on pages 85 and 86.

Let go of worry. Turn it over to a Higher Power then forget it.

Reflect on yourself and others in your life. Reflection is healthy – maybe some answers will begin to take shape.

If you are dealing with an old, unresolved issue, reframe it and release the negative charge.

Begin to do things that make you happy.

Learn to live in the present moment. Fear is rooted in the past and future

Learn To Become A Priority
It's All About Me!

O n the path to healing, with a focus first and foremost on getting well, other people and other things may have to take a back seat until your healing journey is well launched or perhaps over. This doesn't mean you put the rest of your life on hold but it does mean you have to make yourself a priority. This can be a difficult step for the "pleasers" in the world. If you are one of those selfless people who give and give and give, find it uncomfortable to receive from others and have a "to do" list a mile long - that doesn't include anything that directly benefits you, then you may need to read and re-read this chapter. A successful healing journey requires that first you do what is best for you and your body - everything else comes after. Whew, what a novel concept!

We have all heard the expression - you have to "walk the talk". That means demonstrating to yourself and others that you are doing what you say you're going to do. Doing so, then, illustrates in a very concrete manner that you have made healing a priority. Now, you might say, "Of course my healing is a priority -

I'm reading this book, aren't I?" Yes, but there is a difference between interest and intent. That difference is the action you take and how and when you take it.

In total healing, part of the challenge is to be willing to make the tough choices. That might require saying "no" or not giving in to requests from family and friends to do something counter-productive. It might require change: breaking old, damaging habits that are not beneficial during this period. It might also require more personal discipline. Finally, it might require finding alone time to reflect and receive the messages needed to continue your journey successfully.

Healthy Self-Esteem And Self-Love

The ease with which a person is able to become a priority in her or his life can be directly linked to how healthy that person's self-esteem is - in other words, how much they love and value themselves. The subject of self-love is one of the most important parts of this book and unquestionably, the most complex. Most people, if asked, would say they love themselves - yet, their behavior might not demonstrate that fact. We all know that kind of person. Take for example the relative who has been diagnosed with emphysema but cannot quit smoking, the diabetic who won't stop drinking, the neighbor who has just had a triple by-pass and is too stubborn to eliminate saturated fat from his diet - all these individuals would make the changes needed to stay alive, if they valued themselves *enough*. It may look like a lack of self-discipline, most often it is a lack of personal motivation and deep inside they just don't believe they're *worth* fighting for. For these individuals it would be difficult for them to admit a lack of self-love and that is because maybe it is hard to recognize it.

One classic example is one Dr. Bernie Siegel shared in his book *Love, Medicine & Miracles*. "Consider, for example, Sara, a woman who came to me with breast cancer a few years ago; she was smoking when I walked into her hospital room. Her action clearly stated: "I want you to get rid of my cancer, but I'm ambivalent about living, so I think I'll risk a second cancer." She looked up sheepishly and said, "I suppose you're going to tell me to stop smoking."

"No," I said, "I'm going to tell you to love yourself. Then you'll stop."

She thought for a moment and then she said, "Well, I do love myself. I just don't adore myself" (Sara ultimately did come to adore herself - and stopped smoking.) It was a good quip, but it exemplified an important problem many people have with themselves. Self-love has come to mean only vanity and narcissism. The pride of being and the determination to care for our own needs have gone out of the meaning."[14]

That case study perfectly illustrates what I mean. Self-love eludes the individuals who don't have pride in themselves or have the personal strength to care for their own needs. It is self-love that keeps a person fighting for wellness. It is self-love that allows a person to recognize needs in the first place and push for their

---

[14] Bernie S. Siegel, M.D., *Love Medicine & Miracles*, (New York: Perennial Library, Harper & Row Publishers, 1998), 66.

fulfillment. It is self-love that makes it possible for a person to value his or herself.

People can be loved by their family, mate and friends and not love themselves. Such people can be admired by associates yet regard themselves as worthless. These people can project an image of assurance and professional confidence that fools virtually everyone and yet secretly tremble with a sense of their own personal inadequacy. These people can fulfill the expectations of others and yet fail to fill their own; win every honor, yet feel they have accomplished nothing; be adored by millions and yet wake up each morning with a sickening sense of fraudulence and emptiness. To attain "success" without attaining positive self-esteem is to be condemned to feeling like an impostor anxiously awaiting exposure.[15]

Healthy self-esteem is not as prevalent as we might imagine. It took years for me to realize who I was as a person and the gifts I possessed outside of my professional accomplishments. Others never seem to get there. It can evade the magnificently beautiful woman with incredible wealth and material possessions who is too insecure to express herself authentically, the man with a thriving business and community prominence who is intimidated by strong women, the female corporate leader who indirectly manages thousands of people, but constantly has to prove how smart she is to others. The insecurities and inadequacies are everywhere we look because we all have baggage, we all have a past and most of

---

[15] Nathaniel Branden, *The Power of Self-Esteem* (Dearfield Beach: Health Communications, 2001), 37.

us haven't taken the time, on a personal level, to learn to truly love who we are.

One of the ways to begin developing self-love is to begin to think on your own. Not just rehashing what you have heard or read and not doing or saying what will please others. On this journey, this opportunity will be available over and over again. You will be doing things others won't understand. You will be acting on beliefs you have other's may not support. You will be thinking independently and making choices that differentiate yourself from others. The more you can keep true to what you know is right for yourself and your body, the greater respect others will have for you - regardless of what they may tell you to your face - and the stronger your self-respect will become. That self-respect will translate directly into self-esteem and into self-love.

Narcissism And Self-Love

Narcissism is self-love. Webster's New World Dictionary gives the primary definition of narcissism as: self-love; excessive interest in one's own appearance, comfort, importance, abilities, etc. That doesn't seem so bad for a person facing personal survival, trying to build self-love and nurturing ones self to facilitate healing. Narcissism, therefore, is the perfect prescription.

Although it has a bad rap, narcissism is sometimes an extremely necessary role for us as we work to develop a strong sense of self. Giving ourselves a new image - a new hairstyle, new clothes, perhaps even a new body shape from personal training -

indicates that changes are also occurring within us.[16] Such change is healthy and nurturing.

How do we develop self-love by becoming more narcissistic? Well, if you use caring for a child as an example, we all know that love often develops in the process of caring for another. Everyday tending to a new baby or a new romantic relationship brings a deeper attachment and a stronger love. It is the same for developing a stronger love for ourselves. The more we care for and nurture ourselves, the stronger the love will grow. Here are a few ideas you can begin to use for yourself to speed up the process. Some will be easy, others may require help through books, tapes, seminars or counseling sessions, and some won't appeal to you at all. Select those to which you can relate and begin to incorporate them into your life. The key is to develop a habit of taking care of your body and nurturing your soul.

> Spend a few extra minutes in bed when you wake up. Take your time getting up, use this time to think positive thoughts about the day, do an affirmation, do visualization or express your gratitude for your progress. Or, simply roll over and go back to sleep.

> Put on some make-up and fix your hair every day if you are a woman and take a bath or shower with a little lotion after. This improving how you look will make you feel better about yourself. The ritual of grooming is a nurturing exercise. Men groom, too, in a slightly different manner.

---

[16] Caroline Myss, Ph.D., *Anatomy of the Spirit*, (New York: Three Rivers Press, Harmony Books,1996), 190.

Once a week, take yourself on a date. Go someplace that you love, alone - a movie, rummaging through a book store, browsing in a pet store or sitting in the park. Spend at least an hour enjoying your company.

Become a priority in your life. Think of yourself more and begin to do things that bring a smile to your face and make you happy.

List the accomplishments you are most proud of in your life. Spend a few minutes reviewing the list. Dwell on each one and savor the feelings of pride for a job well done. Self-pride is very healthy.

Buy yourself a wonderful new robe - even if you are a man. Something soft and yummy to wrap yourself in at the end of the day; feeling something against your skin that is pleasing and very soothing, too.

If you are depressed or down in the dumps, go to bed. Curl up in a comfortable position and hug yourself. Sometimes even a slow rocking motion helps give comfort. Hugging is good; you deserve that, as well.

Buy yourself a doll or a stuffed toy that makes you happy - that may be a stretch for you gentlemen but maybe just framing a picture that brings happy, joyful memories and putting it next to your bed that you can gaze and smile at before you drift off to sleep.

In the process of falling asleep at night, take slow deep breaths and become centered. Realize that is where you will find your strength. Find comfort in that feeling.

Listen to music you love in the car - even at home.

Begin getting a massage routinely.

Identify a feeling within your body that makes you uncomfortable. When it occurs over and over, notice the source and eliminate the cause - either gradually or totally. Drop the friendship, reconsider or reinvent the marriage, make changes in your job or begin working on your attitude and reactions to others. Perhaps it's as simple as no longer watching the 10 pm news before bed. Don't subject yourself to stressors that upset you over and over again. You deserve better.

Smile more at others. They will smile back.

Treasure your alone time. Learn to go within for strength and comfort.

Get a pedicure - or give yourself one. Yes, that applies both men and women.

Laugh more. Go see silly movies, read the comic strips or watch funny sitcoms on television. Find humor in life.

Learn to forgive your parents and love them in spite of their faults. Practice forgiveness with others, too - including yourself.

Ladies, have a slumber party with a couple of girl friends - yes, even at your age.

Appreciate your daily rituals of beauty - brushing your hair, putting on lipstick and mascara, keeping your nails nice. These nurture and baby your body; do them slowly and with love.

Share your talents with others in need. Volunteer to be a hugger at the local children's hospital nursery, stuff envelopes for the abused children's shelter benefit, send $25 a month to adopt a starving child in a third world country or volunteer your services to coach Little League baseball, soccer or Pop Warner football.

Identify major obstacles you had to overcome in your life. Make a list of them and give yourself credit for coming through them all.

Look at next week's calendar. Move all the appointments for an afternoon or entire day. Play hooky and see a terrific movie.

Reintroduce physical passion into your life. If your illness has taken your focus off love making, begin again. Share yourself with the love in your life - in a new way. More lovingly, more slowly so it feels good to *your* body.

Go to the health or self-help section of your favorite bookstore. Browse. When you see a book that calls to you, buy it and take it home. It is the book you should be reading.

Buy a dog and begin experiencing unconditional love.

Stay up later than usual one night.

Fix yourself a treat. Lots of peanut butter and jelly on a rice cracker, a scoop of gourmet gelato or a ripe luscious fresh peach.

Find something fascinating on TV, an archaeological dig in Egypt, a documentary about African wildlife or a religious teacher talking to her followers. Spend an hour on a unique adventure.

Make a list of the talents with which you were born. The ones your parents or teachers commented on. Also, list the skills you have learned in your life since. Realize how much you have to contribute to the world, your neighborhood and your family.

Be grateful each day for the improvement in your health. Welcome light and love into your life.

Learning to love ourselves begins by taking time just for us. Time alone; time without others. Our illness gives us a reason to nurture ourselves and to develop a stronger self-love and spirituality. This makes time to correct negative attitudes and eliminate fear. Amazingly, the more self-love develops, the less you will need illness in your life.

The simple truth is, happy people generally don't get sick. One's attitude toward oneself is the single most important factor in healing or staying well. Those who are at peace with themselves and their immediate surroundings have far fewer serious illnesses than those who are not.[17]

In Neale Donald Walsch's beautifully written book, *Conversations with God - Book I,* there is a message within that helps make my point. "Blessed are the Self-centered, for they shall know God. It might not be a bad goal in your life to know the highest part of your Self, and to stay *centered* in that."

"Your first relationship, therefore, must be with your Self. You must first learn to honor and cherish and love your Self. You must first see yourself as worthy before you can see another as worthy. You must first see your Self as blessed before you can see another as blessed. You must first know your Self to be holy before you can acknowledge holiness in another."[18]

---

[17] Bernie S. Siegel, M.D., *Love Medicine & Miracles*, (New York: Perennial Library, Harper & Row Publishers, 1998), 76.
[18] Neale Donald Walsch, *Conversations With God - Book 1,* (Charlottsville: Hampton Roads Publishing, 1995),126.

In case you still have doubts about becoming more narcissistic, let me give you insight from Caroline Myss, Ph.D. and her book *Anatomy of the Spirit*. "This last stage in developing self-esteem is an internal one. People who can maintain their principles, their dignity, and their faith without compromising any energy from their spirit are internally evolved: people such as Gandhi, Mother Teresa and Nelson Mandela. All three of these people were, incidentally, thought to be narcissistic during some stage of their development. Mother Teresa, for example, was almost forced to leave two religious communities in her early days because her vision of service to the poor was much more intense than her sisters could abide. During that time she was thought to be self-absorbed and narcissistic. She had to go through a period of deep spiritual reflection and when the time was right, she acted on her intuitive guidance."[19] You, too, will find your strength from within and begin listening to your intuitive guidance - being self-absorbed in the challenge of wellness. Find a reason bigger than yourself that will propel you to a new level of self-discovery and self-love.

Learning To Say " No"

In demonstrating that we will do what is best for us regardless of what others may think, we may have to take a stand. If your body needs sleep you must be willing to go to bed, even if others are still up watching television. If you are hungry you need

---

[19] Caroline Myss, Ph.D., *Anatomy of the Spirit*, (New York: Three Rivers Press, Harmony Books,1996), 191-192.

to eat, regardless of the time of day - even if others aren't eating. If you require certain foods yourself, you must be willing to fix yourself something different than what others around you might want - without guilt. If you are overly stressed with a particular activity in your life, you have to be willing to say no to that - at least temporarily. You must think of yourself first - before you worry about making everyone else happy.

Now, I have earned the right to criticize individuals who rarely think of themselves first since I was an honest-to-goodness, card-carrying member of the "everyone and everything before me" club. In my early years, I had the perfect role model to teach me the art of selflessness, my mother. She was a remarkable woman, who was considered by some to be the neighborhood saint. She cared for her friends, wounded animals and the hoards of visitors who trekked out to Arizona for a change of climate. Her back door was always open and she always had time for her friends and neighbors - to listen to their problems and never pass judgment. She sat and was patient regardless of what she still had to do or how poorly she felt. She suffered the symptoms of her disease, also rheumatoid arthritis, in silence and always did for others without complaining and without caring for herself. She died twenty years too early.

The lessons she taught me about self-sacrifice were instilled very young. I was taught to think of everyone except myself, lived with a mother who withheld compliments and praise because that would surely give a child a "swelled head" and was not encouraged to reflect on myself or my goals, at all. I was in my twenties before I began to realize that I actually had strong likes and dislikes. It was only then that I began to take charge of my life. ing selfless is a hard habit to break.

When constantly taught to serve others and think of others first, developing a healthy self, setting personal goals, and picking good partners becomes more difficult. This is especially true for women raised in the 50's and 60's many of whom grew up with the Cinderella Complex. We actually believed Prince Charming was coming to rescue us and we'd ride off on his white horse and live happily ever after. That man would be our savior, our salvation. A lucky few young ladies were taught self-reliance and encouraged to pursue their dreams but the rest of us waited for that knight in shining armor to arrive.

A weak self-esteem is not only limited to women with the Cinderella Complex, it also appeared if we were raised in a household full of emotional abuse. It also happened if we were unattractive, overweight, late-bloomers or skinny kids who had painful adolescence and teenage experiences because of how we looked. It sometimes happened because one parent or another favored other siblings and we were aware we weren't the "darling". Sometimes if our parents got divorced, it triggered a sense of guilt and sense of worthlessness - because as a kid, of course we were to blame. Needless to say, a large number of children moved into adulthood carrying with them emotional baggage and an enormous lack of self-love.

So, if you are one of those and came through your childhood and into adulthood by not saying "no" very often - and were grateful just to be included, you can relate. In those days, we went along and tried to please. We didn't speak up, we didn't set realistic limits and we didn't stick to the limits we set. We never thought of ourselves first - because we didn't think of ourselves much at all.

Let's say, however the picture I've painted is totally foreign to you. Let's say you had a splendid childhood, achieved all your goals and married well. Then later in life, you became a parent and developed a wide circle of friends - maybe even social standing in the community. You volunteered, ran a business, were successful in every hobby you undertook and others envied your life. Making yourself a priority might still be difficult because some people with very full lives fall into the habit of 'running'. Sort of a gerbil-in-a-cage routine that grows and grows and one day takes over your life. Your calendar takes precedence over everything. Is that you?

Whichever you are, I'll still bet if I asked you to give me a list of what concerns you most on a daily basis, the list would look something like this: your work on the job or climbing that corporate ladder, having a successful marriage or making your current relationship work, being a good mother or father to your children, spending enough time with your parents or caring for them now that they are older, improving your golf game, organizing an upcoming holiday event and getting all the presents (that you haven't shopped for yet), visiting your in-laws often enough, monitoring the remodeling project in your house, planning an event at home to pay-back friends who have had you over. When you look at your priority list, I'll bet you're at the bottom, if you're on the list at all.

Taking care of everything and everyone else is a wonderful and noble thing - but not at the expense of ourselves. Sometimes being selfish can be good - especially when you are struggling to get well.

I knew a woman once whom I really admired as a mother. She had wonderfully behaved, happy children. And, I asked her what her secret was to raising such a well-adjusted brood. Do you know what she said? "It's them, or me." Her response startled me because it seemed so out of character for her.

She was a loving person and she was gentle and compassionate but she also had balance in her life. She didn't give into every one of her children's demands, even when they were very, very young. She had household rules that included schedules for eating and sleeping so mom could actually have time to clean the house and take a bath. To her, that behavior wasn't selfish; it was merely survival.

Thinking of ourselves does not have to be a foreign concept even if your beginnings set the tone for different style of living. If you were like me, you may have been taught that thinking of oneself was a bad thing - and that thinking of oneself *first* was reprehensible. But, when you are ill, priorities need to change - not just for a day or two, but for the entire time you are getting well. Hopefully, that will then become a habit you will carry into the rest of your life.

A profound lesson is taught every time we fly. It is illustrated over and over when the flight attendant of every commercial airline in the air announces, "If there is a change in cabin pressure an oxygen mask will drop from the ceiling. Grab hold of the mask and press it firmly to your face, pulling on the side straps to tighten the mask. Secure your mask, first, before helping any small children." This, dear friends, is a lesson in survival and common sense for if you don't take care of yourself, you can't take care of others.

For individuals, who have forgotten themselves in the process of being a good employee, a good boss, a good spouse, a good mother or father and a good friend, being stricken with a major illness can be a wake-up call for our own nurturing. In this process, we must learn to care for ourselves, to get in touch with our needs and to begin to focus on the signals our miraculous bodies give us. We can't do that unless we are on our 'to do list'.

A unique perspective, once again, is provided by Neale Donald Walsch in his first book, *Conversations with God – Book 1*, when he states, "God asks only that you *include yourself* among those you love. God goes further. God suggests - recommends - that you put yourself first." This was meant in context of putting yourself first in the highest sense, which is not selfish but is necessary and simply means doing what is best for you without causing harm to another.[20] So, if you want good health - begin to develop habits of caring for yourself that will help perpetuate your good health - not weaken it. Begin by thinking of your health and yourself, first, before trying to please others, maintaining the same old bad habits or succumbing to the pressure of family or friends.

Welcoming Alone Time

Not surprising, when something like a debilitating or life threatening illness hits, our priorities change. We are *forced* to

---

[20] Neale Donald Walsch, *Conversations with God - Book 1*, (New York: Hampton Roads Publishing, 1995), 132.

think of ourselves: how we hurt, how little energy we have, or what might happen as this condition progresses. Our families begin worrying about us, too, and watch often helplessly at how we are coping. If the problem is painful or debilitating enough we can be faced with plenty of alone time.

For the first time in your life, you have a real opportunity to look at yourself, your health, your lifestyle and your relationships. From time to time this is necessary but for those of us who have continually pushed past logical assessment times every few years, illness like we're facing will force the issue.

Years ago I heard a commencement address in which the speaker advised the graduates to take time to hear God's whispers, because if we don't, there will be louder requests, finally yelling and eventually what she called "earthquakes" in our lives, to get our attention. If we are experiencing severe, chronic or life-threatening illness, we have obviously missed the whispers. Those whispers were gentle, loving messages from a Higher Power telling us that we are important, that change is needed in our lives, that perhaps there are things we are doing that are not beneficial for us, or that we need to pay more attention to ourselves. When those whispers become "earthquakes" it's still not too late to re-think our priorities, to spend more time getting to know and understand ourselves or perhaps get more connected spiritually.

Illness doesn't always reveal only the positives, however. Sometimes with real time to reflect - we find parts of our life horribly depressing. It is at times like these when we want to curl up alone in bed and hug ourselves while we drift off to sleep.

Learning to go within and comfort ourselves is a very positive by-product of the illness that has beset us. We may begin to love and nurture ourselves more, maybe for the first time in our lives. Focusing on us, remembering we are important and beginning to put ourselves and our health above all else are essential for total wellness.

If symptoms of your illness haven't already slowed you down, then you need to make additional time needed for self-reflection. It's one thing to realize why you need more time for yourself, it's quite another to take it. Here are a few suggestions to make the process of finding more time a little easier:

Work fewer hours. If you're used to overtime, cut back to a 40-hour week. If you run your own business or have flexibility with your hours, start an hour later each day or end your day an hour earlier.

Divide up household chores. Ask your family to pitch in. If you cook, have someone else clean up. Send out more of your laundry or hire someone to iron. If you live alone, stretch out weekly chores to every 10 days or 2 weeks. Do less.

Say *no* to any social functions that are not absolutely and positively necessary.

Put outside activities you don't simply *love* to do on hold. Take a time-out for a few months.

Sleep later in the morning.

Go to bed earlier at night.

Send the children to Grandma's for a visit more often than normal - multiple days, if possible.

Turn off your phones every once in a while.

Cancel unnecessary appointments.

Then, when those precious extra hours appear, the first thing to do is to use them to bring peace and contentment into your life. Peace and contentment cannot co-exist with a mind full of useless clutter or worry. The answer to that is meditation.

Learning to Meditate

Meditation is really not that mysterious; it is merely keeping your mind empty and staying in that peaceful, calm place for as long as you can. So, when thoughts drift in, don't focus on them just let them drift out. Keep your mind motionless and still. Find a book on meditation or buy a tape; meditation is learned through practice. There are a number of ways to begin to quiet your mind.

My favorite is to take slow, deep breaths and follow your breathing with your mind - in and out, slowly. That rhythm, that focus on nothing but the sound of your breathing, will keep your mind still. Then, later, whenever you find yourself with a few quiet moments use that time to decompress. Try to clear your mind, again. As thoughts enter your mind, gently push them out so you are blank. Enjoy the quietness of that space. Eventually you will have more mental peace and less worry. The past disappears and the future is unimportant - you begin to get focused in the moment. If you are more comfortable using quiet music and visualizing a peaceful setting, use that method. I am personally not as fond of using mantras but you will be drawn to the method best suited to you.

As Deepak Chopra, M.D. says, in his book *Journey into Healings*, "When we experience pure silence in the mind, the body becomes silent also. And in that field of silence, healing is much more efficient."[21]

Quieting the mind is also an effective process to help manage pain. I found that when I was in the most acute pain, the more active my mind was, the more intense the pain became. The more quiet and still I remained, the more it eased. Having a peaceful, still mind has other benefits, too. Those familiar with biofeedback techniques will see the similarity. It is the first step in becoming truly centered, being able to listen to our body's signals and learning to live in the now.

Back to Valuing the Alone Time

Private time or alone time also allows you to explore other options that exist for your healing - options you may have never considered before. Buy new books, learn and explore. Select ones that call out to you or to which you are drawn. One book at a time to start, but certainly books on holistic healing or alternative method by any of the prominent healing messengers I have mentioned earlier. Use your quiet time for personal growth.

Alone time is also a great time to listen to audiotapes or watch videos. Most popular, self-help authors also have these tapes available. I found myself buying various audiocassette series and listening to them while I drove to my office and back. It was a

---

[21] Deepak Chopra, M.D., *Journey Into Healing* (Harmony Books - 1994) p 97

refreshing break from the routine and a way to keep focused on the wellness I was seeking. I did not find that any one tape was the panacea for me, but rather, I found something of value in every one of them - a little here and a little there, all of which I would eventually incorporate into my healing ritual.

Alone time is also perfect for prayer. Taking time to be grateful for each bit of progress you experience and for the messages you are routinely sent.

Old Habits Die Hard

All too often, in the face of a major illness, people struggle to keep up a tough exterior and drive ahead doing exactly the same things they did before they became ill. They don't realize that this illness might be a wake-up call to slow down or make changes in their lives. They think they can just push through it. Well, this is what I share with individuals who attend my workshops on healing, the definition of *Insanity:* "*Doing the same thing over and over and expecting a different result.*" That pretty much sums up the need for change - if we want a different result in our lives. But, to some of us change can be a real struggle.

In my particular case, I had built a successful advertising agency at thirty years of age, the first woman owned agency in Arizona. I was proud of my accomplishments, in general, but everyday brought newer and bigger challenges. As an entrepreneur, I had to learn the basics of business and as a young advertising professional, I was still learning more about my trade. There was stress at every turn.

The advertising business is a business of deadlines, which causes plenty of pressure in its own right. And, as a small business owner there were often things I was forced to do because of a lack of human or financial resources. So, I did them regardless of the stress it might have produced. Everything else in my life came before me: my clients, my employees, my son, my husband, and my parents, one of whom was dying of cancer. I was also concerned about my husband's children and making their time spent with us memorable. I was luckier than most because I had a housekeeper but managing her and trying to devote quality time to my family when I consistently worked 70 - 80 hour weeks was an ongoing challenge. We took very few vacations and when we did, we tried to include all the children, so the times away from the office weren't necessarily restful. I also felt stress and suffered from guilt for not having time to be the kind of mother, wife and friend I wanted to be. There simply wasn't enough time for everyone. And, there certainly wasn't *any* for me.

Those of us who have been through similar situations realize that there is a routine in being that busy constantly. You could compare it to being on a treadmill, and the treadmill is winning. The worse part of it was the guilt I suffered and the regrets I had - for the quality time I needed to spend with my only child, for the thank you notes I wish I had written but never did, the entertaining I longed to do but never had time to organize, and the friendships that had suffered from neglect because of my business and lifestyle.

Becoming ill forced me to stop my old patterns. My rhythm changed; weakness and exhaustion gave me more alone time. Joint swelling and stiffness forced me to stay at home or be an observer rather than a participant. Pain helped me learn to become totally still. Because of my condition, I spent more time by myself and began to break old, counter-productive habits that kept me too busy, for me. Because now I had to do less, I began to make choices and select only the activities that were most important to me. I began to become more discriminating. I had no choice.

Learning Personal Discipline

In the course of change - another characteristic will emerge - personal discipline. That, my friends, is the process of honoring the changes before you and not falling back to your old, counter-productive habits and lifestyle.

Your changes may be many and varied. Your diet might change. You might begin to think about what you should eat and what you shouldn't. You might have to pass on a glass of wine because you are rebuilding your immune system. You begin concentrating on how you feel; you begin to pay attention to your body. When you begin to get tired, you have enough sense to go to bed. When you can't do any more, you simply stop. And, guess what? The world doesn't come to an end. Instead we learn how to make better choices, we learn to determine what we need versus what we want, and we begin to discern what works and what doesn't. Illness is a very good teacher.

Saying no, doing something different than others are doing, paying attention to the needs of your body all require discipline. You can do it - you will want to do it - as soon as you begin to see progress you will be empowered by doing it. It is almost like the excited feeling we get when we step on the scale and realize we have lost two pounds. The diet becomes a challenge we know we can meet. Every bit of progress we experience propels us forward with more enthusiasm and energy. It is the same with your healing; your discipline will become stronger with every step in the right direction.

Thoughts to Consider

Welcome the opportunity to nurture yourself – you deserve it.

Gandhi, Mother Teresa and Nelson Mandela were all thought to be narcissistic during some stage of their development.

Even on airplanes we are reminded to take care of ourselves first.

Your healing journey comes first – everything else comes second.

Truly happy people generally don't get sick.

Meditation is not that mysterious – it is merely keeping your mind empty and staying in that peaceful, calm, neutral place as long as you can.

Insanity is doing the same thing over and over and expecting a different result.

Steps to Take

Make yourself a priority by putting yourself and your wellness first.

Reflect on the way people treat you – this
can reveal if your self-esteem
needs bolstering.

Begin to form your own opinions – whether you share them with others or not.

Begin taking care of your body and nurturing your soul (see the list on pages
102-106).

Take time just for you
(see the list on pages 114 and 115).

Practice saying 'no' – politely.

Use your new alone tine for personal
growth. Read a book, listen to a tape or
watch a video.

Slow down – stop the treadmill and take
time for yourself and your healing.

Learn to meditate and to clear your mind.

Begin experiencing living in the
present moment.

Forget yesterday and tomorrow – your
power lies in the choices you make
right now.

Use this newfound time to reflect on your priorities and to understand yourself and the
relationships that surround you.

Commit To The Journey
There Is No Silver Bullet

A nyone who undertakes a holistic healing journey and has never experienced one before will need some explanation about what to expect and what not to. Because the process is so different from conventional medicine, managing expectations was part of the reason for this book. Had I known twenty-five years ago how my healing would unfold, the entire journey would have been much easier.

First, in a holistic healing journey there is no quick fix. You might have guessed that by the name holistic, that there is total healing on multiple levels. The holistic process is, then indeed, a journey. This can be tricky for the individual who expects immediate gratification in all facets of his or her life; a person who wants everything right now. It is also tough for the individual who is overstressed, impatient and not tolerant of any process whatsoever. Finally, those who have been totally conditioned by the allopathic model of treatment, which taught us to believe that a single office visit, a simple prescription or surgery will fix everything on the spot. If you are any of the above – you will need to adjust your expectations. Holistic healing takes time. The payoff: healing is permanent.

Here is a recap on how it basically unfolds: you make a statement of intent, first. Then you wait for the answers and all will come at the perfect time and in the perfect order. You act upon them as they appear to you - so the second and third steps happen simultaneously. But, because the healing is on three levels - the spiritual, emotional and physical those answers can jump around among the three categories as needed to ensure lasting and complete success. The complexity dictates much more time than a couple office visits or one hospital stay. It could take months or years. As long as there is continual improvement and as long as your body is becoming stronger, naturally, it doesn't matter how long it takes.

There Is No Quick Fix

A silver bullet or quick fix is typically reserved for band-aid-type cures that are never effective in the long term. Those symptomatic fixes rarely get to the root cause of an illness or keep it from returning. That is why so many chronic conditions exist. A person keeps running back to the doctor over and over for symptomatic relief but years later the person is still sick.

The use of conventional medicine also advocates the gatekeeper approach in terms of one physician controlling care, whereas the holistic healing process is dramatically different. We are used to finding a doctor and trusting that one person to give us all the answers or refer us to specialists on occasion. What happens with a holistic healing journey is that there will be many sources of help along the way, often simultaneously, and each one will provide expertise in his or her own arena with no one practitioner having all the answers. A patient takes what is of value from each source and selects those sources typically on their own.

In alternative medicine it is perfectly acceptable to move around a little: to stop going to someone, to make a change to another practitioner or to add others to the mix. That could mean you have several practitioners - all for different reasons. Perhaps a masseuse you use routinely for lymphatic stimulation and circulation, a naturopath for general work, a chiropractor for skeletal adjustments and a Jungian counselor for dream interpretation. You could add acupuncture, some Chinese herbal medicine, a homeopathic practitioner or you might see a holistic MD. Because this process can be self-directed, you will learn as you go and you will always be led to helpful decisions regarding your health. Guidance will come when you are ready for the next step and throughout personal responsibility will play a key role.

Taking Responsibility

The most tragic part of the allopathic regimen is the belief that it is your doctor who heals you. That is not true. As was discussed earlier, on a physical level, it is a person's body that heals. On the emotional and spiritual level healing occurs at the soul level. Healing does not come from some external source. In holistic medicine, practitioners take time to learn about the person, learn about that person's body and then both patient and practitioner do what they can to help the body heal itself.

There was a brilliant Canadian physician and medical historian named Sir William Osler, who once said the outcome of tuberculosis has more to do with what went on in the patient's mind than what went on in his lungs. He was echoing the sentiments of Hippocrates, who said he would rather know what sort of person has a disease than what sort of a disease a person has.[22]

Hippocrates, the father of modern medicine, was born in 460 and died about 377 B.C.; he was credited with freeing medicine from superstition. Although all doctors take a Hippocratic oath before they begin practice I doubt whether they are familiar with all of Hippocrates' beliefs. The idea of preventive medicine, first conceived in *Regimen and Regimen in Acute Diseases*, one of Hippocrates books, stresses that diet and the patient's way of living could influence his or her health. Physicians today and we as patients tend to ignore the details of diet and lifestyle in our healing. That is where personal responsibility enters the picture.

What does taking responsibility really mean? When our bodies are in top form they are miraculous instruments. They kill germs, destroy viruses and bacteria, defeat cancer and zap other assorted critters that might invade or be housed in our bodies and they do that on a daily basis. That is the job of our immune system. But, when our immune system is weakened or compromised - these intruders can take hold and temporarily overtake our systems. Over time we learn that it is the choices we have made in our life that weakens or strengthens our immune system. Past transgressions always show up later.

---

[22] Bernie S. Siegel, M.D., *Love Medicine & Miracles*, (New York: Perennial Library, Harper & Row Publishers, 1998), 2.

As we look at our health and look at the shape our bodies are in today, it doesn't take a rocket scientist to determine that we may have done some damage to ourselves in the early years. The overworking, the overeating, the overwhelming stress, the drinking and smoking might also have been factors. For some, it was even drug use in the 60's or later. Our abuses chipped away at the magnificent machine we were given, little by little, until our bodies were weakened and are now beginning to give out.

Years of too little sleep may have taken its toll especially if we crammed for exams for a number of years, dated and partied until all hours of the night or worked multiple jobs with too little rest. We probably also ate lousy food and developed bad recreational habits including limited exercise or a yo-yo program of weight loss and we are now seeing the result. If we didn't learn how to release our emotions when things got too bad, if we stuffed and stored our feelings, if we were young and ignorant and invincible - today we're probably paying the price.

So here you are in trouble. If you can admit choices you made might have contributed to the weakening of your body, you have just taken the first step toward getting well.

If you can weaken your body you can also strengthen it. Accepting responsibility is the first step to taking control of your healing.

It's Not My Fault - It's In The Genes

Some people try to excuse their illness based on a family history of one condition or another. Genetics are no excuse for poor health. Some people are very lucky and come from a strong gene pool, but most of us have a number of chronic or life-threatening ailments somewhere in our family tree. There are potential problems we have inherited from one distant relative or another including heart disease, cancers, arthritis, and sometimes even more exotic strains lying-in-wait in our bodies. Yes, many of us were blessed with destructive genes.

Still, even if a person might have a predisposition to a condition, it does not guarantee they will actually contract it, especially if their natural defenses are in good working order. For example, we all have cancer cells floating around within our bodies but we don't all get cancer. One of the jobs of our immune system is to scan cells in order to recognize and eliminate those that do not belong there; it routinely weeds out the malignant cells. We have developed this defense over the course of our evolution and it works - unless we have weakened our immune system in one-way or another.

In my own case, there was a strong genetic case for my eventual rheumatoid arthritis diagnosis. On my maternal side, there was an uncle and aunt both severely crippled with rheumatoid arthritis, a female cousin currently suffering with it and my biological mother, (you recall my being adopted at birth) has osteoarthritis. Yet, I have been able to regain my health and live pain free and drug free by keeping my immune system strong enough to keep this weakness from surfacing in my body. Leukemia is also within the family lineage with an uncle who died from it and a cousin who is currently struggling with the disease.

Genetic weaknesses can be prevented if we are aware of those conditions and don't encourage that pre-disposition through our own reckless behavior. At the risk of oversimplifying, if we have a propensity for diabetes, we'd watch our weight and make sure we get plenty of exercise. If we are prone to heart disease, we wouldn't load up on saturated fats. For most conditions, simply learning how to rid our lives of stress and not generate more can be beneficial. Basic education, common sense and a desire to preserve our bodies is what is needed to ensure good health.

Even if illness strikes, there are a number of things we can do to help ourselves recover. The control we have regarding our health comes mainly from the choices we make every day. And, no one but us makes those choices.

Healing Is Cumulative And Progressive

As you are exposed to many different teachers and coaches on your journey you will notice that each practitioner will impart something valuable. It may be advice, a recommended treatment, or a supplement to take. All along the way you will pick-up bits of information that you will add to your "routine" to help your body improve. You'll know which ones are right because your body will immediately respond and you will see some degree of im-provement. When there is no improvement - you might rethink the treatment, supplement or practitioner and probably remove it from your regimen.

Holistic healing is a cumulative process. So, if a certain vi-tamin or mineral is recommended and you notice a slight improvement - say 5 percent - continue with it. If acupuncture is something else you experience and you jump another 20 percent with this modality, keep that too. Now, you are at 25 percent. Let's say you begin another method that helps another 25 percent - now you are at 50 percent. You are headed in the right direction. When you improve, you don't quit the regimen. Too many people, the minute they start improving, quit what they are doing that helped get them there. A big mistake. You continue with what works because it is those things that are keeping you on track. The goal is to get as close to 100 percent as you can.

I began taking a certain level of Vitamin C nearly 25 years ago; I still take roughly the same level today. There are a couple more supplements I am consistent with and others I add on an as-needed basis. I see certain practitioners for some treatments and have modified my lifestyle to generate less stress. I have my 100 percent program in place and it works beautifully. As my life situation changes, I modify it a little, but basically the team of providers and remedies is in place and I have learned how and when to use them.

With each experience your body will judge its value. Some providers will give you advice about what you should do with your lifestyle or nutritional choices still others will provide direct remedies. Some will provide spiritual resources and emotional tools. Odds are you'll receive something you need on your journey from every experience you have.

Over time, it will become possible to build up a regimen of therapies and treatments as well as practitioners that work for you. That is why alternative methods are best used as early as possible, while there is time for the process to work and when your body has not been ravaged by devastating drugs or radical surgery. That doesn't mean you have to begin at the first diagnosis; even toward the very end - one can achieve results. It just becomes tougher to do when you wait because of the toll unsuccessful medical treatments will have already taken on your body. With surgery, for example, the body becomes so distracted trying to heal after the surgery - it cannot focus on fixing itself. With chemotherapy, radiation or other powerful drugs, the immune system is rendered helpless or has been totally shut down so it could take longer to restore its healing potential to finally attack the disease it was originally designed to. Since you're relying on your body to do the healing, you'll want it to be as healthy as possible to begin.

Time Is Your Friend Not Your Enemy

Time isn't something that you manage on this journey – it is what it is. Progress will also not happen on your timeline so forget trying to control that, either. With every visit, with every new treatment or remedy and with every experience along the way – something new will be learned. The magnificent reality of a holistic healing journey is that not only is the timeline set according to how quickly you are able to learn, absorb and apply each lesson but the answers will come in the perfect order to compliment the chemistry of your body and the receptiveness of your mind. The timing becomes irrelevant.

As long as you are improving, you are moving in the right direction and the process is working. Again, because we are dealing with the complexities of holistic healing and working with the spiritual, emotional and physical factors - those elements will come to you as you are capable of receiving them. The more open you are and the more receptive, the more rapid your healing. Some folks are ready and grasp the physical part of the healing journey but the mental and emotional or spiritual pieces may take a little longer. It doesn't matter in which order your progress comes - it will come together in the perfect order for you.

To reiterate once again, the longer window of time you have to heal from your illness - the better for alternative treatments. That is why alternative methods are ideal for anyone with a chronic condition. There is no excuse for living with a dis-ease that goes on and on and on and on and on. Critical illnesses can also be overcome but it becomes more challenging with your diagnosis reveals a very short window. When there are only days or weeks available, it is best to begin with allopathic treatments. Alternative care can become supplemental to build-up your body and try to repair the damage done during the allopathic process. Then when the aggressiveness levels out - a transition can more easily occur, if that is your choice.

My father was diagnosed with lung cancer in 1980 and told he had a maximum of six months because of his inoperable tumor. His doctors gave him radiation to help the tumor shrink but doubted it would do much. It didn't. A stubborn man and a smoker, my precious father said he would follow whatever I suggested to help since I was so devastated at the thought of him leaving us. He quit smoking and began Vitamin C therapy, which in those days didn't involve intravenous methods that could have accelerated his results. He took Vitamin C orally with a maximum dosage of 10,000 units daily (practitioners are using higher doses today). Within three months his tumor had shrunk to 35 percent its size and amazed his doctors. His radiation had stopped long before this with unnoticeable results. This progress was achieved without any major diet adjustment and also in spite of a few puffs on a borrowed cigarette from time-to-time. As he began to see some improvement, his confidence increased about his crazy daughter's methods and he relented to try a trip to Mexico for laetrile injections, which was the popular alternative therapy at that time. Daddy was still pretty weak and couldn't drive so Mom drove their camper down to the border where the two of them visited an alternative clinic. Mom learned how to change their diet of 40 years and she tried her best to cook foods that would be less stressful for his body to digest.

Four months later, on a Saturday morning I heard my door-bell ring and there stood my father and mother. Daddy had a smile on his face, having driven back from Mexico all by himself. He was much stronger and had regained a little of his old zest for life. We found a woman in his town to give him the laetrile injections (a nurse who agreed to help) and he continued his treatment at home. His slow but steady progress through the end of that year (10 months from his original diagnosis) had already defied the medical prognosis of death by six months. He was still improving, but, my daddy was old school, stubborn and impatient. He still didn't feel 100 percent, hadn't gained much weight and couldn't go fishing, continue his routine of smoking and drinking like the good old days and couldn't play cards until late at night like he used to.

Even though it had taken a number of years for my father's body to become weak enough for this cancer to appear, he just didn't want to wait for the measured improvement. My father was not a fighter and had never been. He had really tried the therapy just for me and although he was remarkably better and his tumor was minute compared to where it was, he wouldn't fight any longer. He quit everything - the diet, the laetrile, the Vitamin C and he continued to smoke every once in a while - even later with Hospice care at home and oxygen in his room (he'd smoke in the bathroom with the window open and door closed). He passed away in late April, 1981.

My father lasted 14 months - more than double the original prognosis and could have completely recovered had he been patient enough but he was a man who resisted change; change that meant no more smoking and drinking until he was completely recovered - and probably not the smoking - even then. He was living with a new diet he wasn't used to and he was in a recovering mode, which made him "different" than his friends. He hated that. Had his faith been stronger, had his tolerance for change been greater and had he been patient with the timing, my father might have lived to see his great grandchildren, whom he would have loved. Somehow, living under those conditions wasn't worth it for him.

To completely heal, it can take weeks, months or years. One just has to be patient and realize that if you are stable or even slightly improving - you are headed in the right direction. So, patience is a must. We must also remember how long it took for us to break down our bodies in the first place - enough to allow the disease to take hold. If your body took years of abuse you can't expect miracles in a few short weeks.

Healing On The Physical And Emotional Levels

Understanding the mind-body-spirit healing model is not difficult. Especially if one takes it, isolating the focus to one specific disease, and dissects the process so it is easier to grasp. In the case of my rheumatoid arthritis, on the physical level, for example, I was initially being treated to relieve joint swelling and pain by a rheumatologist. Of course, the pain didn't totally subside but it was dulled dramatically because the drugs reduced the inflammation in my joints causing the pain. Had I been satisfied with relieving just that, I never would have been free of the eventual crippling and debilitating symptoms of this disease. Later, surgeries would have removed the calcium deposits from my joints but the ugly crippling would have still been present. On top of it, I may have had face swelling from all the cortisone prescribed and suffered from a host of other side-effects from taking the many drugs. Side-effects like irritable bowel syndrome, colitis, depression, irritability and other symptoms I regularly experienced.

So when I made the change to holistic healing, my focus was getting to the physical root cause of this condition, which was an auto-immune disease and involved a T-cell malfunction. I could only truly be rid of the RA when I got my immune system and those pesky T-cells functioning more normally. That was a tall order and much too complex for me to try to figure out all by myself - so I decided to leave it to my body to heal and ask to be guided to the right answers to make sure that marvelous machine of mine was given all the tools it needed to perform masterfully on the physical aspect.

On the emotional or mental level there were also root causes with which to be dealt. These were often more complex. Once you identify some of your emotional blockages you will find messengers bringing you advice or suggestions to which you will relate. It may be a friend who shares a similar story, a guest on Dr. Phil or Oprah that sounds eerily familiar or an article in a magazine you feel compelled to read dealing with the subject. Absorb the information and then try to apply the lessons you have learned to your own life.

With leukemia, it was equally complex but I had simple benchmarks to watch on the physical level: my energy level, my white count and my lymph count. I could have been content with fixing those with the Vitamin C therapy and a couple other reinforcing supplements I used but eventually it would have returned in that form or some other until I fixed the final *real* problem. That *real* problem began at the emotional level as I also read in Louise Hay's book: brutally killing inspiration, "What's the use?" lack of joy or lack of circulation of ideas. I had addressed the "unfinished business with my family of origin." Caroline Myss defined in her book. The real trigger was the giving up - the "What's the use?" portion that set the wheels of this condition into motion. I finally dealt with all three, which is the reason I had such remarkable, steady results.

In retrospect I was able to identify exactly the time when I subconsciously "gave up". I had just experienced a number of days anger directed at me by my husband that left me emotionally exhausted and spiritually bereft. The reoccurring event, this time, was devastating to me. I was so full of pain I was numb. The one salvation was the existence of my son, my only child and someone I adored. At that time, he too, seemed to emotionally abandon me. He was getting married and was captivated by his wife's family, which pulled him away from us more than usual. Because I was so emotionally vulnerable at the time, I actually felt as though I was losing him to another family. Whether this was real or imagined, it didn't matter. It was real to me at the time. It wouldn't have been so devastating had it not been the fact that these two people were the closest to me in the world - since all my other immediate family was gone. I can remember saying to myself, "I can't take the pain. I don't want to be here anymore." It was only a split second but the grief was so real and both emotional attacks hit simultaneously, which was just too much for me to handle. I had given up.

That was in February, 1999 and by April I was so tired I could barely function. I thought it was my workload, a huge presidential fundraiser I had co-chaired in Phoenix and a couple other significant projects I was working on for a nonprofit I cared about then. Month by month I got weaker and felt worse. By August I went in for a check-up and in September I had the diagnosis. It was this simple: I said it; my body heard it and then delivered what I asked for.

Realizing what triggered the onset of the leukemia and doing the emotional work to clear the old family of origin issue, I had only to find my joy. That happened months later in the spring with the birth of my first grandson. With that my healing accelerated and I knew the last emotional element had been satisfied and the leukemia would never return. The joy search was fascinating for the goal was to find it again in my life. When I had searched for joy I didn't know where to begin. I looked at old photos to try to identify when I was truly joyful. I was happy. I was excited. I was optimistic and positive. I as even content at times but none of that was true joy. Then little Charlie was born and the moment I saw that angel in his father's arms - and he looked exactly like my son, Jon, had looked when he was born - I was overcome. This was, indeed, joy. Once I experienced that feeling again, I was able to find joy in other parts of my life: my friendships, a glorious sunset, the magnificent nature all around me and in daily experiences I had taken for granted. After that, my healing began making lightning progress.

One never knows what will trigger a feeling like that. To myself, I call dear little Charlie my "Joy Boy". Since then, I have been blessed with two other beautiful and very special grandchildren who have magnified that joy enormously. Just a tiny dose of Charlie, Jack or Lucy makes my life true bliss.

The Spiritual Level

On the spiritual level you will find healing, too. For me, the natural progression of my healing on the other two issues and the time it took to eventually get well provided the platform for spiritual growth. You, too, will find a connectedness that you never dreamed would occur. Some people are already connected solidly in the spiritual arena and so trust and faith will come easily. For others, it will take time and will unfold throughout your journey.

You should look for progress in the quiet time, the silent time, the alone time you experience. When you begin to quiet your mind and learn meditation - you will be able to listen more intently and to read your body more readily. Quite often then your Higher Power or Higher Self will talk to you, very often through spontaneous thought.

As you surrender and become humble in this process, it will be amazing what develops as a result of all the intense emotional work, physical adjustments and work you do at the soul level. I opened up my creative side, got clear about my purpose, and found peace and contentment I never felt before. Probably the most remarkable results were the intuitive gifts that appeared; those shocked me. Much of what I describe will happen to you, too, as you pass through a similar wondrous time.

Through this remarkable journey, you may begin to see and then become overwhelmed with gratitude for a life that does not have to be a struggle at all. All the answers are there. We simply have to ask and they come - sometimes in odd forms - but who are we to judge?

Thoughts to consider

A holistic healing journey and the process
for conventional medicine are
totally different.

Holistic healing happens on three levels: the
physical, the emotional and the spiritual.

There is no silver bullet.

Healing is cumulative and progressive.

Not one person will direct you to all
the answers.

In alternative medicine it is perfectly fine to
access more than one practitioner.

Your doctor does not heal you – it is your
body that heals.

A genetic predisposition is no excuse for
poor health.

Time is your friend not your enemy.

As long as your body is improving, you are
moving in the right direction and the
process is working.

A cure may be only temporary, healing
is permanent.

Steps to Take

Realize that you played a role in your body's
present condition.
Take responsibility.

Begin to build a regimen that will work
for you.

Keep what works – discard what doesn't.

Don't set expectations – go with the flow.

Surrender and become humble during the
process. You don't have all the answers

Make Healthy Decisions
Toss Excuses Out The Window

I don't know which seemed more overwhelming – the initial choices the world of alternative medicine presented or the adjustments I needed to make every day in order to really commit. It is all daunting if you are used to your doctor making all your decisions for you and not doing more than take a pill a day. Thinking about the magnitude of all those choices can be very frightening. That is why I remind you - it may seem like that proverbial "elephant" but the choices are really fewer than you think. The goal is to follow along and limit your thinking, period.

You are not expected to be savvy about every alternative option available, how they work, or if any one makes sense for you. Remember, this will be 15 percent intellect and 85 percent intuitive and feeling. So, it's fine if you want to read on the Internet or buy a few books to educate yourself from time-to-time to learn more, in general. But because there is so much to learn because you need to begin your journey quickly - you can read and learn as you go. Any other preparation is not necessary.

To make the process less frightening, I want you to remember you really only have three overall choices to make. The first is to decide where you are headed - your focus. The second is to embrace the journey wholeheartedly without fear and to actually begin by visiting an alternative practitioner. The third is what you do on a day-to-day basis in terms of putting yourself first, exercising self-discipline and maintaining a healthy attitude. With everything else, you will be guided.

Regarding your first choice - your focus: just remember to keep your eye on the ball and stay directed on becoming healthier and on seeing continued improvement in your condition. Do not become the LUPUS lady and stay buried in your disease by looking it up continually on the Internet, talking about it incessantly, learning every detail and nuance and wallowing in self-pity. Let it go. It is what it is and you are going to get over it very soon. Stay focused on becoming well and how being well previously felt. The first choice is the most important choice of all, and the most simple.

The second choice, where to begin or, more specifically, what practitioner to try first is only partially up to you. If you did what was asked in earlier steps, the Universe or God will provide those opportunities. You need only to act on them. You will not control the process or the timeline, so being overwhelmed by the choices is needless worry. You need only to remember to act and learn as options come to you. Some people may feel, however, they want to make the first step themselves. If that is the case with you, you will get help in this chapter on how to accomplish that.

The third and final category of choice *is* yours. Those choices involve the real details of healing: the attitude with which you approach this journey, the choices you make in your day-to-day routine, what you eat, what you think and say and how much you learn as this process unfolds.

Choosing Whom To Trust

As was discussed earlier in this book, conventional medicine is a wonderful system for diagnosis. So, keeping a good family physician or internist in your stable of resources is a must. Routine checkups are helpful and if you are noticing very odd, recurring symptoms you can't understand, go see what your doctor says is wrong. Just remember not to buy into the prognosis if it is limiting. If it *is* limiting, you may want to look elsewhere for help. Also, if the medical community, through its treatment protocols, has been unable to facilitate satisfactory progress with your issue, if it has been unable to diagnose your condition at all, or if you have been referred to at least one specialist unsuccessfully - it could be time to try the alternative route. Remembering what conventional medicine does well and what it doesn't do well makes it much easier to decide where to place one's trust.

Now, the question of trust really surfaces when it comes to the field of alternative providers. Who should you trust and who shouldn't you? Here is where it actually becomes simpler. You don't have to *totally* trust any of them - any more than you should totally trust your allopathic doctor. You should ask questions, learn on your own and try what is recommended - watching for the results your body will reveal. Whatever your treatment, you should not experience any negative side-effects. If you do, your body is telling you it is not happy with what you are doing. Be open to each option put before you, try it and see. If it works - even slightly, keep it - and add others as they come to you.

Real trust should be conferred upon a Higher Power and your body. You trust the Higher Power to deliver opportunities to you and you trust your body's reaction to what you are experiencing. Pretty simple. It will become obvious whether or not you continue with a treatment or remedy. A healing journey is a process that connects us more strongly to our spiritual selves.

As you become more in-tune spiritually, which will happen as you surrender and are willing to be led, you will eventually begin to trust your intuition, as well. You will find we are all healers and we were all given by God, or a source greater than ourselves, a multitude of gifts to use.

Your Immune System Will Be Key

The immune system controls our body's healing system on a physical level. It can be the key to recovering from many diseases and conditions that range from fibromyalgia, chronic fatigue and infections to cancer. The more we learn about this incredible, internal system - the more we can take control and make better choices to help our bodies heal.

Our immune system has an enormous number of conditions related to its function. You can tell some by the names they are given: auto-immune diseases and immune deficiency diseases, for example. Auto-immune diseases occur when the immune response becomes misdirected and focuses its aggression against our own body's tissues or organs. In other words, our immune system goes haywire. When it does, it can affect the nerves, joints, endocrine glands, connective tissue or muscles through a variety of different diseases. Even though we may also have a genetic predisposition to conditions like multiple sclerosis, rheumatoid arthritis, myasthenia gravis, lupus or others, it is usually emotional trauma, physical stress or an infection of some sort that triggers the onset of these diseases.

There are also diseases called immune deficiency diseases, which occur because our immune system becomes deficient or weakened. The most notorious are HIV-AIDS, chronic fatigue syndrome and Epstein-Barr, which are viral-based diseases or conditions that have been allowed to progress. An immune system that is temporarily weak may also set us up for a host of other, viral-based conditions such as: the notorious hantavirus, bird flu, mononucleosis and West Nile virus. Less traumatic, but equally stubborn can be the common cold, respiratory virus, influenza, and herpes simplex and herpes zoster. The list for viruses might also include infectious rabies, measles, warts and mumps.

A weakened immune system is also susceptible to bacteria-caused conditions that can be air or food born, cancers and conditions caused by parasites, fungi or microorganisms. We can be protected from all of these with a healthy immune system that destroys those culprits before they can destroy us. None of the conditions I have mentioned stand a chance if our internal defense mechanism is in top form. Conventional medicine has had little or no success offering cures for these diseases even after spending billions of dollars in research over the years. Neither has it trained its doctors in preventive measures to help people strengthen their immune systems on their own.

Are You Sure Cancer Isn't Different?

No, cancer has a direct relationship to the immune system, too. One of the jobs of the immune system is to scan cells in order to eliminate any that do not belong in the body. As I mentioned before, this surveillance system weeds out malignant cells. If cancer appears - it is not because we caught it from another person or from something floating in the air - it is because there has been a significant failure in our internal surveillance system. Cancer only attacks us when our immune system becomes suppressed or depressed and our routine "surveillance mechanism" breaks down. If there is cancer in your body, even in its earliest stages, it represents a significant failure in your healing system.[23]

According to Andrew Weil, M.D., "If someone has cancer, conventional treatment can do very little except offer surgery, radiation or chemotherapy." He also states, "Only the first procedure makes any sense at all, for removing the cancerous growth, if possible. The second two are crude treatments that will be obsolete before long. If someone chooses radiation or chemotherapy, there will be damage to their immune system. The question in selecting treatments like these is whether the damage done to the cancer justifies the damage done to the immune system."[24]

---

[23] Andrew Weil, M.D., *Spontaneous Healing* (New York: Alfred A. Knopf, Inc., 1995), 267-269.

[24] Andrew Weil, M.D., *Spontaneous Healing* (New York: Alfred A. Knopf, Inc., 1995), 267-269.

Cancer remains a dreaded disease and puts fear into the hearts of nearly everyone receiving the diagnosis. That fear is one of the emotions that weaken the immune system and that in itself is counter productive to the healing process. According to many, attitudes that generate a feeling of powerlessness can compromise the immune system by robbing a person's body of the energy it needs to sustain good health. So, the quicker we decide not to let the disease overtake us and instead that we are going to overtake the disease, we will begin to regain our energy or power and begin to strengthen the system designed to fight this condition. Because our immune system is so critical to our health, it is to our benefit to learn what makes it strong and what makes it weak.

The immune system is made-up of a magnificent network of cells and chemicals. It is your body's defender. It identifies, tracks down and destroys biological troublemakers that enter our bodies whether it's bacteria from a cut or scrape, a chronic virus, a pesky germ or aggressive cancer cells. Our immune system is what masterminds the attacks on diseases before we get them. This miraculous system manufactures a host of internal pharmaceuticals and dispenses them to the appropriate part instantly, stopping those internal invaders dead in their tracks. This exquisite internal pharmacy makes the right medicine, for the exact time, for the perfect target organ - with no side effects. It works for us 24/7. This wondrous defense system can prevent us from getting everything from the common cold to cancer and to fight off afflictions as frightening as AIDS, if we keep it strong.

What Weakens And Strengthens The Immune System?

One of your key goals - in order to protect yourself from cancer and any other disease - should be to keep your immune system functioning properly. To educate yourself about what makes your internal defense system strong and what makes it weak, doesn't have to be as technical as it sounds. Once you understand the basics of holistic healing, the rest can come from common sense.

Below is the list that I assembled over the years to help me make better choices in day-to-day living. This list doesn't tell you how to achieve the result, it does outline in general terms what weakens and what strengthens the immune system, according to my experience.

WHAT WEAKENS AND STRENGTHS THE IMMUNE SYSTEM		
	Weakens	Strengthens
BODY	Physical stress such as environmental pollution, loud noise and chemicals	Calm, peaceful atmosphere
	Excess candida albicans	
	Drugs – illegal, prescriptions, caffeine, tobacco, alcohol	No drugs
	Chemicals in foods – dyes, preservatives, aspartame	Healthy, fresh or frozen food
	Food allergies or sensitivities	
	Lack of sleep	Plenty of rest

	Weakens	Strengthens
		Replenish/enhance body nutrients (vitamins-minerals-other substitutes)
MIND	Fear, anger, resentment, guilt	Love, forgiveness, compassion, gratitude
	Attitude – negative	Attitude – positive
	Stress – emotional	Release daily emotional stress
		Release stored, negative emotions
		Mental therapies-affirmations, visualization
		Self Love
SPIRIT	Hopelessness	Faith
		Trust

Keep this list handy and refer to it everyday - it will help guide you about questions to ask your holistic coach or practitioners, give you hints on areas to work on and offer topics for further study.

There are a number of other tips, more tactical in nature that should also help. Remember to laugh, pray, think positively and live a balanced life. Take deep breaths, warm baths and spend time with close friends. Limit antibiotics and drugs in general, take supplements - especially Vitamin C, Vitamin E and B complex. Don't eat processed or refined foods - especially processed sugar. Eat fresh or frozen vegetables -without pesticides, if possible. Keep good bacteria in your intestinal system - acidophilus can be a good supplement for that, plus foods like dill pickles, sauer-

kraut and miso soup. These are suggestions you might want to jot down on post-it notes to place on your bathroom mirror, kitchen refrigerator or wall in your office.

Thoughts to Consider

You will learn as you go – preparation is
not necessary.

Whatever treatment you try should not produce negative side-effects.

Your immune system is critical to
your healing.

The lifestyle choices you make can influence your health – for the bad and for
the good.

Steps to Take

The attitude you adopt throughout this journey – can make it pleasant and an adventure
– or can make it drudgery.

Ask questions, learn on your own and try
what is recommended.

Trust your Higher Power to guide you.

Remember what strengthens and what weakens the immune system on pages 148 and
149. Only do what strengthens it.

Make sure you have a good family physician
or internist in your stable of providers.

You are in control of which doctor and
which method of treatment you accept.

Realize Illness Is A Gift
Don't Fall Victim To The Victim Trap

W hy did this happen to me? A common question from those faced with chronic illness or a life threatening disease. Although we may ask the question over and over it generally goes unanswered. No matter how hard we try, we can't seem to figure it out, our friends can't give us a response that quiets our desperation and our doctors can't enlighten us in a way that gives us comfort, either. For most of us who are physically suffering, this pleading mantra is more a cry to be rescued than a search for the truth. However, to those of us who have accepted personal responsibility, realize we may have contributed to the existence of this condition in the first place, and rejected the concept of merely being a victim of all of this - our illness can become a tool for growth and a catalyst for change.

It is easier to become personally responsible if a condition is directly related to lifestyle. Therefore, change in physical habits will keep these conditions from getting worse or reappearing later. To over simplify, lets take the obvious such as quitting smoking or drinking if you have a disease related to the lungs, throat or liver. Weight loss will also make sense for those with diabetes and heart disease. In cases that appear simple, lifestyle changes can make a huge difference - but are never the entire story. Also on a physical level, we may have a functioning deficiency that needs attending with nutritional supplements or bad lifestyle habits that involve lack of sleep or too much stress which may have taken their toll and left our immune systems in a wreck. Changes in those situations are logical and often a snap to understand.

What is harder to understand is what illness might be teaching us on the emotional or spiritual levels. There are messages here as well. That is why the mind-body-spirit link is so magnificent and the core of holistic healing. Illness is not just a physical condition. It is much, much more and if we don't deal with the aspects on all levels, the odds are the illness will return in one form or another.

If you are like me and believe that we, alone, create all situations in our lives, then it is easy to accept that our illness is there for a reason. Some of you may be more fatalistic and believe everything in life happens as a result of an overall plan, not of our own. In that case, it is feasible to accept our illness is also there for a reason. If neither of those ring true for you, perhaps you can accept that subconsciously we might create a situation in our lives that helps us in ways we cannot help ourselves on a conscious level. Illness might, then, be one of those situations. If the illness you are experiencing is not for the purpose of helping you leave this earth, then it is here for another reason.

Getting Well Again, a classic bestseller about revolutionary life saving self-awareness techniques, by O. Carl Simonton, M.D., Stephanie Matthews-Simonton and James L. Creighton reveals a startling list of five categories they found from a survey of their patients. These benefits seemed to be the most frequently listed when asked how their illness benefited them. Look at this list of five benefits illness delivers to some people. See if any of those have ever applied to you - or currently apply. Be honest with yourself and even if you can't relate to some or most of these, be kind to yourself when the realization hits you. I have taken these categories, which are numbered, and expanded upon them with paragraphs under each, to help you see how the reason might be applicable to you.

1. Receiving permission to get out of dealing with a troublesome problem or situation..

This can be permission to "hide" and to avoid dealing with something uncomfortable or something with which you don't yet have the tools to deal. Yet, the beauty of illness is that through this process, you may be able to receive the time you need to strengthen yourself in that area of your life where you are weaker or not well equipped.

2. Getting attention, care, and nurturing from people around you.

This is a much more significant statement than it appears. Your illness may be providing you the opportunity to gain attention, care and nurturing from others but it also could be providing you the same opportunity to gain attention, care and nurturing from yourself.

For most women, illness is the only time they take to pay attention to themselves. This is unfortunate. It is also one of the many reasons, in my opinion, besides connecting spiritually; illness exists - to give us the opportunity to grow in self-love. That can only come from taking time for ourselves, respecting ourselves, realizing we are deserving of wellness and loving ourselves unconditionally.

3.   Having an opportunity to regroup your psychological energy to deal with a problem or to gain a new perspective.

Illness can be a much-needed "time-out" that gives us the opportunity to reassess a situation we are in. Sometimes simply by recognizing there are situations that exist with which we have few or no tools to effectively resolve, we can see where we need to grow and improve or where we need to change direction.

If not stimulated by a particular event, this can be a time to reflect on our values and priorities, a time to discard the values or priorities that no longer apply or have a positive purpose in our lives and to embrace those things that now have more meaning. By realigning those priorities and values we make different and better choices going forward.

4.   Gaining an incentive for personal growth or for modifying undesirable habits.

Once a significant disease hits, it is simply easier to quit or modify undesirable habits. The need for personal growth is not always as quick to recognize. Often, through the time illness takes from our lives, we gain the "time-out" to be more reflective.

Personal growth can include an attitude change, emotional clearing or spiritual growth. Without the illness we may have never been aware of the need that exists and we may have never had the additional time to focus on that challenge.

5. Not having to meet their own or others' high expecta-
    tions.[25]

Although it can be a much-needed excuse for non-performance; it can also be a time when we take back our power. This can be a time when we learn to answer to ourselves first, before others, and a time when we become more realistic about our expectations for life. It can be a time when we become more forgiving of ourselves and of those around us.

In a society where we are so stressed and pushed for time that feelings and emotional needs often take a back seat, disease can fulfill an important purpose. It can provide a way and the time to become aware of a significant issue and to work toward solving it consciously. In giving you an "out" or an "escape" this break that illness presents also gives you the time to grow and to reflect. First should come the realization that you needed the time-out. Second should come the gratitude for giving you time to solve the problems in your life, which might have contributed to your disease in the first place.

Your Illness As A Messenger

Besides giving you the time you need to take a closer look at yourself and your life, your illness can point to the areas that need the most work. The key to identifying the changes that need to occur in your life lies in your ability to accept the premise that your illness, itself, is your messenger.

---

[25] O.Carl Simonton, M.D., Stephanie Matthews-Simonton, and James L. Creighton, *Getting Well Again,* (New York: Bantam Doubleday Dell Publishing, 1992), 133-134.

If you can begin to recognize the benefits, which have occurred in your life, as a result of your illness, then you can start to unravel the complexities of your individual path of learning. To begin, take a sheet of paper and on the left side, make a list of the benefits you have received as a result of your illness. To the right, begin to list the characteristics you might need to improve or the areas for personal or spiritual growth which could result from the benefits list you first created.

For example: if you have found your illness gave you an opportunity to gain nurturing from others, it might mean you should examine your relationship with those other people. Are they healthy relationships? Are they ones that need repair or ones you should walk away from? Do you nurture *yourself* enough? Do you make time for your needs or express them to others in a way people can understand? Are you only intellectualizing your needs and not acting upon them? Are you doing enough in your life to promote your own self-respect and self-love?

Life is full of answers if we are open to receive them. Our bodies themselves provide us answers every day. So do the situations that occur in our lives. Don't go through life with your eyes shut or your mind locked into paradigms that stifle personal growth and development. Illness helps us re-examine our lives, our values and our priorities. For many of us, it provides the opportunity to create a new and more meaningful life. If we approach our illness as a curse or a burden, we miss the messages being sent. We miss the opportunity to clean up old emotional baggage, rectify self-destructive habits and realign our priorities to make our lives richer and more full.

156

The gift of illness is the key to unlocking the answers for healing, which occurs on the emotional or mental and spiritual levels. Once you accept this premise, you will begin to look for the "gifts" your illness is delivering to you and through that list of benefits, you'll be able to short-cut the personal discovery that is needed to stimulate your emotional and spiritual growth.

Your illness will be your teacher. It will help guide you through a learning that will not only heal your body but can heal your spirit, too.

The Gift Of Enlightenment

Illness gives us the gift of time so we can do the growing that's necessary. It slows us down so we have time for the process at hand. It helps us focus on ourselves so we can begin to respond to our physical, emotional and spiritual needs.

Your illness gives you a chance to get in touch with yourself in a more meaningful way; a way you would never have attempted by living your old habits and routines. This illness broke your routine and gave you an intervention - a chance to change.

Your illness has given you a second chance to become enlightened. The dictionary definition of enlighten is: "to give the light of fact and knowledge to; reveal truths to; free from ignorance, prejudice or superstition". What a gift.

Yes, illness presents us with many gifts and this break in your routine offers the opportunity to fix the things that were broken, learn more about yourself and evolve in a more positive way.

Now that you are in control and recognize the wonderful opportunity before you, seize the moment and begin that positive change.

Thoughts to Consider

Seeing illness as a misfortune can hinder the healing process.

Your illness is here to give you time to fix things which need fixing in your life and in yourself.

The gift of illness helps us unlock the keys to healing on both the emotional and spiritual levels.

Illness can be a good teacher.

Steps to Take

List the benefits your illness has given you. Those benefits might give clues to areas you need to strengthen or improve.

Look up the emotional root cause of your condition. See how that might apply to you. Do affirmations to correct those shortcomings.

Learn to apply what you have learned. Take action.

Examine your relationship with others and yourself.

Examine your spirituality. Do you feel content, loved and connected to a Higher Power on a daily basis?

Gratitude Propels Progress
A Little "Thank You" Goes A Long Way

B y this time you should have a pretty clear understanding of the mind-body-spirit connection in healing. You should also recognize that the mind/emotion part of the formula is much more complex than just exercising positive thinking, which many individuals tend to believe is the crux of the emotional piece. In order to successfully address this element it is important to be in touch with one's emotions, which is a challenge for many, but really is pretty simple.

How emotions play a critical role becomes much clearer if you can relate negative emotions to stress generation. Begin with fear, one of the two base emotions - the other being love. From fear stems a host of other reactions, including anger, jealousy, criticism, resentment, guilt, control, hostility and selfishness. Without even understanding the biochemical or biological implications of living with fear, long term, it is not difficult to see how this state could easily generate internal stress and weaken the immune system. Now magnify that stress with the stress caused by the behavior we create while living in those negative emotional states. How positive emotions strengthen our immune system may be a little tougher to grasp. One of the easiest ways to get the picture is to try to see how the power of emotions sets the tone for our lives.

The emotions and attitudes that dominate our personality also begin to dictate what life delivers to us. If we sow the seeds of generosity, light-heartedness, forgiveness and optimism, those are the flowers that bloom. If we sow the seeds of anger, pessimism, criticism and resentment, then those will be what proliferate in our life. This is the law of attraction applied. We attract what we think, believe and demonstrate. So, selecting the right attitude helps shape the results we experience.

The good news is we have the ability to choose which emotions we evoke. That might be tough for individuals who have lived a long time bathing themselves in unhealthy emotions. But, it is never too late to learn and there is one easy place to begin.

Becoming Grateful

Gratitude is an extremely powerful healing emotion that is central to accelerating one's healing experience. It's impossible, however, to be grateful for things in our lives if we're moving too fast to notice them. So, before you learn about how gratitude works, you have to learn to slow down.

One great way to slow down is to meditate for a few minutes every morning becoming more centered and creating a more peaceful feeling within. I always ask that the day flow effortlessly and peacefully. I then approach the day much calmer and less rushed. Such a process also helps a person live in the present moment, so you can appreciate a warm, gentle breeze, the birds chirping first thing in the morning or the smell of orange blossoms on the way to your car.

Being "in the moment" one is able to see the obvious in a more appreciative way; nearby bushes and grass appear a more vibrant green, the blue of the sky becomes more electric and the movement of tree branches and leaves become more rhythmic. Yesterday doesn't seem as important and tomorrow seems a long way off. You are enjoying exactly where you are and therefore you are able to appreciate the greatness of life.

Once we take time to look at our daily lives it is easy to identify parts of it to enjoy; significant elements for which we might actually be grateful. Sarah Ban Breathnach, in her book, *Simple Abundance, A Daybook of Comfort and Joy,* recommends keeping a gratitude journal. She says that by consciously giving thanks each day for the abundance that exists in our lives, we will simply not be the same person two months from now. We will also set into motion an ancient spiritual law: the more you have and are grateful for, the more will be provided to you.

As Sarah recommends, every night before going to bed, write down five things that you were grateful for that day.[26] Maybe it was the smell of cinnamon rolls as you passed by a shop at the mall. Maybe it was an unexpected note you received from a friend or maybe you were grateful that you were able to locate your lost dog. Instead of focusing on the fact that the dog irritated you by

---

[26] Sarah Ban Breathnach, *Simple Abundance: A Daybook of Comfort and Joy* (New York: Grand Central Publishing,1995).

running away, be happy you found him. But then, if the day was an all-around stinker - and, some are like that - you can simply be grateful the day is over.

The power of gratitude extends past the power to strengthen your immune system. Its ability to evoke the universal law, that Sara mentioned, is equally powerful. To illustrate that point, just imagine one day you give your little child a toy. He takes one look at the toy and throws it down on the ground. The second day you give him another toy and this time your child turns his nose up, drops it and walks away. On the third day, with yet another toy you've provided, your child doesn't even bother to open the sack for several hours, it just lies there on the floor. With an attitude like that, how likely are you to give that youngster another toy in the near future?

Conversely, you are friendly with the little neighbor girl who is delighted with the flowers you let her pick from your yard and she thanks you every time she does it. On her birthday, a simple card from you brings a warm smile and a hug. When you give her some of your junk jewelry for dress up she squeals with delight and the first time she wears it she runs over to your house just to show you how pretty she looks. You see a grateful child is one for which you can't wait to do even more.

We are all children, in a way, and being grateful for the progress we make in our healing or just being grateful for having a good day helps deliver more of the same. Being sincerely grateful produces many wonderful by-products because you begin to change your focus from living in a world that's half-empty to living in one that's half full. You begin to focus on the positives. Sara's idea of a gratitude journal is a marvelous one to remember.

By reflecting on the things you were most grateful for at the end of the day, you conclude each twenty-four hours on a positive note. What a wonderful place to be before drifting off to sleep.

Acknowledge Your Progress

It is also possible to focus gratitude on a particular subject for a particular result. Being grateful for the positive, productive relationship you have with your children will encourage you to recognize your children's good qualities and helps those qualities expand in your perception. The result is an even more positive, productive relationship. What someone focuses on expands.

If you believe in God and prefer relating this to God's generosity, then thanking God specifically encourages even more of the same because, as mentioned before, we are all children of God and the prayers of gratitude we send forth are, in a way, paving the way for even more Divine gifts.

Simply stated, focusing on your progress in healing will create the same response. Seeing the progress, acknowledging it and thanking a Higher Power for what is being given to you encourages more and more of the same.

Give Yourself Credit, Too

At the same time, taking a little credit yourself is also perfectly healthy. In fact it is beneficial for you were not only guided by a Higher Power but you took personal responsibility, took action, made life changes and did everything you needed to in order to help your body heal. You deserve some credit, too.

There is nothing as rewarding as having done a good job and recognizing that fact. It is in the recognition of self where some people fall short. Doing good work or meeting a goal should be a time to celebrate. When you finally reach the desired result because of your actions you "own" the result. It is precisely then - and it is warranted - to revel in your accomplishments and bask in the glow of self-pride.

Instead of being impatient with how slow the progress is coming or the degree of progress so far - be thankful you are continuing to make progress at all and still moving in the right direction. Remember, you are now in control and you and your body are doing this on your own. You are becoming stronger and healthier every day. You are listening to your body for answers, you are more connected spiritually and you have the potential to become totally well - without drugs and their side effects. Each step you take is a positive one - headed in a direction to provide a much-improved quality of life. You are the captain of this ship - and you should be extremely proud.

For each of you who are launching on this magnificent, healing journey - you deserve a lot of credit. But, once you begin you will see that this will be the most productive and meaningful series of experiences ever and the results will amaze you - not only because you will have recovered - but you will have learned and grown in remarkable ways. This, my friend, will be the most significant journey of your life.

Thoughts to Consider

Love based emotions strengthen the immune
system. emotions like gratitude, exhilara-
tion/joy and love, itself.

Steps to Take

Keep a gratitude journal. Every night list
five things you were grateful for during
that day.

Sow seeds of generosity, light-heartedness,
forgiveness and optimism, and those are the
flowers that will bloom for you.

Choose emotions that are positive – that
attitude will help shape the results
you experience.

Acknowledge your progress. Focusing on it
will create more.

Offer prayers of gratitude for what is
working well in your life.

Give yourself credit.

Enjoy the journey.

SECTION TWO

The Extraordinary Benefits
Of a Holistic
Healing Journey

CHAPTER ELEVEN

You'll Find Spiritual Connectedness
No More Feeling Totally Alone

O ne of the most amazing benefits on the path to wellness is the spiritual journey that evolves. It comes automatically. Yet, it is not necessary to be a practicing member of a religion to find wellness, to develop your spiritual self or to find a spiritual advantage along the way. I separated the spiritual part of mind-body-spirit healing because it is so profound and so intricately woven throughout this experience. It begins with having faith of some kind - of *any* kind. Faith that answers might exist some-where. It continues when you exhibit trust in the process. Total healing cannot occur if a person feels hopeless and has absolutely no faith.

Now, I do not mean faith in a secular sense, but faith in general. Whether it is faith in God, in a Higher Power, in the Universe, Spirit, or even in yourself. For holistic healing to work - the two elements that must be present are some form of hope and some form of trust. The rest will evolve as you move forward.

I had not been religiously active for years yet always considered myself very spiritual. I accepted the concept of a Higher Power or God but hadn't reconnected with a formal secular relationship in the last thirty years of my life. My previous religious experiences failed to deliver the environment I needed for my own personal spiritual growth. I was critical of many of the teachings to which I was exposed, especially those based on promoting fear and dependency. For those reasons, I fell away from any organized effort.

Spirituality Surfaces Automatically

I was a number of years into my healing of rheumatoid arthritis and would have assessed myself as 80 to 90 percent well. Even though I had truly mastered the physical aspects of my wellness and I had little or no joint swelling or stiffness, unless my candida albicans flared up because of too much stress or eating the wrong foods too often. I had pain a couple times a year but it was mild and could be managed with two aspirin, a cold pack and ace bandage while I slept. I had learned to strengthen my immune system and these changes in my life improved my health dramatically. I was perfectly happy - but I still didn't consider myself 100 percent well.

It was about that time when I began to notice a shift in the information that was of interest to me. I was now being drawn to more books on spirituality. Books like the *Celestine Prophecy* became fascinating. Marianne Williamson's, *A Return To Love*, Marlo Morgan's *Mutant Message Down Under*, and M. Scott

Peck, M.D.'s *The Road Less Traveled* were stacked on my night stand. Today those books might be titled *The Secret; Eat, Pray and Love; The Purpose Driven Life; How to Know God* and *The Path to Love*, among so many others. New friends also entered my life, all who were on the same spiritual quest. They also wanted to find more meaning in their lives and were becoming more connected to something greater than themselves. We would meet and share books we had read and lessons we had learned. We all wanted to feel peaceful and to have our lives flow effortlessly every day. In retrospect, the spiritual connection and a lack of stress seemed to go hand in hand. We wanted to experience abundance and great health and joy. I had seen glimmers of perfect days and I wanted more.

I began to make the connection between spiritual growth and how effortlessly my life could flow. I realized a peaceful feeling created better health - I wanted to feel peaceful more often. I also realized love and spirituality were connected. I wanted more love in my life and I was beginning to open up to it. The messages that were now coming fast and furiously to me were no longer about stress management and vitamin therapy, they were about understanding and developing more love in my life.

I wanted to meditate more and began to relish my alone time. I wanted to be filled with love and a peaceful feeling as often as possible. I savored the extra half hour when I awoke or the extra hour at night when I went to bed a little early that helped me capture that mood. Those silent times became precious to me and while I quieted myself so I could better set the intention for each day, I found additional messages coming to me. When my mind was very silent I received additional guidance to help me capture the peace I so desperately sought.

I found other methods to help me achieve the tranquility for which I was looking. I was drawn to gems and minerals and began to recognize how their energy supports our efforts not only in physical healing but spiritual enlightenment. I discovered essential oils and found them beneficial, too. I began to use the pendulum I had used with my Radionics machine to access other information I needed. All of which gave me a tremendous sense of security and peace. That peaceful feeling and contentment was becoming just as important as my lack of pain. Each of these tools tapped into my intuitiveness and connectedness.

As I continued to explore other aspects and perspectives on spirituality, I began to find philosophies and strategies, which appealed to me. Therefore, ways to become happier were enhancing my health and ways to become more loving were strengthening my immunity to disease.

As I reflect on that time, the time I recognized that spirituality was truly part of the healing process, I can identify the most significant learning that occurred to me:

I began to live in my heart and not in my head.

I accepted me the way I was. I became less critical of myself and therefore, others.

I found joy in myself - in being alone with me.

It was easier to refrain from thinking negative thoughts such as criticism, competitiveness, resentment, jealousy and especially anger.

172

I released false expectations that made me frustrated and angry when they did not occur. I trusted more.

I shared my joy and wealth with others.

I began to live my purpose and follow the joy. I consistently did more things that made me happy and began to express my true talents.

I loved myself and nurtured myself more.

I put fear aside.

I learned to relax and go with the flow.

Your experience may be completely different. But during my journey, I began to feel closer to God and to feel a true sense of protection and love. For me those feelings came without reconnecting with an existing formal religion, but for others that process may be better suited for you. I found my spirituality and its role in healing when I was ready for it and with that spirituality came a stronger trust in myself.

Although the ritual of attending a weekly service was absent from my life, it was replaced with my own rituals of daily communication with God during my quiet or alone time. Expressions of gratitude, feelings of love and requests for guidance, for me, didn't require certain physical locations or structures. My own gatherings with friends, while reflecting on our spiritual growth, provided the social infrastructure I needed. I could - and did - experience spirituality in a way that was comfortable for me. The catalyst for truly reconnecting with a source greater than myself was my illness and the increased amount of quiet and alone time I was experiencing. The solitude in my life restarted my spirituality and feeling closer to God.

Religion And Wellness

God wants us to be healthy and happy - that is why He gave us the miraculous body he did. Many religions may not teach that directly, but there has always been a link between organized religion and wellness. Larry Dossey, M.D. explains in his book, *Healing Words,* how prayer and spiritual practices have always influenced our physical health:

> The teachings of Mormons, Seventh-day Adventists and Orthodox Jews all include precautions regarding diet, alcohol, hygiene and other health-related behaviors known to favorably impact morbidity and mortality.

> The collective aspect of spiritual practices provide social support, which has been documented as a potent protective factor against illness.

> Rituals such as prayer may trigger myriad of emotions that, in turn, may lead to changes in health by positively impacting the immune and cardiovascular systems.

> The psycho dynamics of faith can be indistinguishable from the placebo effect.

> Experiencing the presence of a healer or healers may foster a sense of belonging or support, which research shows is healthy.

> Being the object of prayer or the laying on of hands or other ritualized activity may stimulate an endocrine or immune response facilitative of healing.

The physical preparations for healing such as meditation, some abstentions and preliminary fasts may themselves be promotive of health.[27]

These findings were affirmed for mental health by the National Institutes of Health physician-researchers David B. Larson and Susan S. Larson who found after surveying twelve years in publication of the *American Journal of Psychiatry* and *Archives of General Psychiatry*, that participation in religious ceremony, social support, prayer and relationship with God had a positive benefit in 92 percent of the cases, neutral benefit in four percent of the cases and negative effect in four percent of cases.[28] Similar findings for physical health, in research by F.C. Craigie and his colleagues, in a 1990 review of ten years of publications of the *Journal of Family Practice*, 83 percent of the studies showed benefit, 17 percent were neutral and none showed harm.[29]

---

[27] Larry Dossey, M.D., *Healing Words: The Power of Prayer and The Practice of Medicine* (New York: Harper Collins Publishers, 1993) 252-253.
[28] D. B. Larson and S.S. Larson, "Religious Commitment and Health: Valuing the Relationship," Second Opinion: Health, Faith and Ethics 17:1, 1991, 26-40. Larson and Larson's teaching module: *The Forgotten Factor in Physical and Mental Health: What Does the Research Show?* (An Independent Study Seminar: Washington, D.C.: National Institute for Healthcare Research 1992).
[29] F.C. Craigie, Jr., D. B. Larson, and I.Y. Liu, "References to Religion in the Journal of Family Practice: Dimensions and Valence of Spirituality," *The Journal of Family Practice 30:4 (1990), 477-80.*

Trust And Connectedness

I was lucky because my religious background and present belief system allowed me to accept there was something more powerful, more knowing and more loving than I. Therefore, when I became determined to help myself, I knew help would be possible. I always felt the possibility of Divine intervention existed in healing, whether it was direct or guided. I wasn't certain how that help would present itself for me - maybe I was just supposed to help myself.

Back then, I did not understand coincidence, I did not understand the power of intention and I did not understand how answers might be delivered to me. The process of the simple law of attraction and in where one places focus, were also concepts with which I was totally unfamiliar at the time. I also wasn't sure how having faith translated into help on my journey. I never thought fervent prayer throughout the day to ask for help and guidance made any practical sense, I was much too practical for that and felt much of this would be up to me.

My experience proved that, at least for me, and after I simply stated my desire and had the absolute confidence God or someone would hear me and help, that is exactly what happened. Maybe it was extreme self-confidence on my part, maybe it was a knowing that answers did exist somewhere, or maybe it was simply the strength of my intention and a willingness to do whatever it took to make that intention a reality. Today, I believe a Higher Power heard me and put in my path all the tools I needed to get the job done. I knew God didn't want me or anyone to truly suffer.

Trust and spirituality are the cornerstones of the healing process and through them you will find tools to help you heal. As you participate in this marvelous journey, your spirituality will be reinforced and enhanced and you will begin to appreciate and marvel in the way answers are delivered to you at precisely in the moment. I believe you will come to realize, as I did, that this is a Divinely led journey.

Even the most hardened skeptic will come to grasp how masterfully the tools for finding wellness work: visualization, affirmations, coincidences and how our bodies communicate with us to attract new methods and to report the results of those we try. Then, in the course of honoring our self-nurturing rituals, offering prayers of gratitude and seeing how effortlessly the flow of life carries us along our path, the power of the connection becomes overwhelming. It is impossible not to feel a sense of oneness; that we are, indeed, interconnected to each other and to a higher source of power.

The "we" factor brings with it an enormous source of peace and contentment. Realizing we are not alone and that we have infinite power and information at our disposal - always - is the core of true spiritual contentment. It was very hard for me to articulate the feeling that results from experiencing a journey like I have been through, even though it had happened several times. Recently, however, I attended a Celebrate Your Life conference in Scottsdale with fifteen hundred others who wanted to gather to hear prominent voices speaking about spirituality, soul purpose and a host of related subjects. As a result of that experience, some of what I heard may help you understand even better than I could convey it.

177

One of the speakers asked attendees of his workshop to look at the words illness and wellness. When you write them one under the other, the only difference are the letters "I" and "we". Then, Michael J. Tamura, in a subsequent yet non-related workshop offered, "It is that separation from the whole or the "we" that encourages disease and stands in the way of truly becoming well." How simple - yet, how profound. Michael J. Tamura, a world-renowned spiritual teacher, healer, author and speaker - even in a field of others at this conference like Deepak Chopra, M.D., Dr. Wayne Dyer, Caroline Myss, Ph.D., Neale Donald Walsch, Joan Borysenko, Ph.D. and James Van Praagh - touched my heart the most and I knew what he had just shared with us was important to share with you.

When the journey to healing occurs, it is the holistic process that makes the spiritual connection and helps you become fear-less. You will see that in the course of this journey - everything begins to make sense. Each step of the way you will begin to expand your thinking by embracing and trusting the unknown, your faith will grow, you will feel more connected to the whole and peace and contentment will flood into your life. To experience that - with or without total wellness - is worth the trip.

Thoughts to Consider

Consider the mind, body and spirit in your
healing and develop all three.

Trust that answers will come to help you –
and they will.

You don't have to be a member or an organized religion to connect with your
spiritual self.

Steps to Take

Remember and use the rituals or practices
that made you feel closer to a Higher Power
or develop new ones.

Welcome new friends who are also on a spiritual quest. They will give you support.

Be open to books or other messengers who
communicate spiritual insight that might
help you heal.

Honor self-nurturing rituals.

Offer prayers of gratitude.

Remember how connected 'we' all are in the
Universe. Embrace that connectedness
with love.

Carve out more and relish your alone time.

Trust. Find a spiritual connection that makes
you feel safe and secure.

CHAPTER TWELVE

You Will Also Learn To Love Yourself More

You'll Be Surprised What This Will Do

T he beauty of holistic healing is that it considers *you* the process. It is not just looking at a symptom and attacking the symptom - patient be damned. It considers the whole. Now, saying that self-love will be a by-product of holistic healing may be a leap for some of you, but, it will really occur if this roadmap is followed, For built into the journey is a process of becoming a priority in one's life. That can't happen without enhancing one's self-love and eventually, boosting one's self-esteem.

It is my opinion that self-love is the critical component to healthy self-esteem and having a healthy self-esteem makes life a whole lot easier. When a person has healthy sense of self they simply make better choices. Those choices will include consideration of oneself and thereby how the action impacts decreased stress. The effect of stress on our health is a given. So, developing self-love, in itself, can be a catalyst to better health.

Since the early 80's, I've been involved with nonprofits and the empowerment of women - not in the sense of "liberation" but in the sense of helping them develop a healthy sense of who they are. Also, having been the programmatic architect of the first comprehensive self-help center for women in the country and watching women's lives change one after another (for several years as CEO of the governing foundation for that particular center), I saw the effects of self-love and self-esteem and how inextricably they are tied.

With healthy self-esteem a person begins to see the world differently; she or he then comes from a perspective of fitting into the picture and when that happens, the choices they make become more personally beneficial. Someone who feels unworthy continually attracts people and situations to reinforce that unworthiness. It is a vicious cycle. So, to break the cycle, one must change how one feels about oneself. Self-love is the beginning. When a person develops a greater love for his or herself, the life choices also shift and more sound decisions are made in that individual's best interest. Specifically, that person selects healthier friends and partners and develops lifestyle habits that reinforce their own value. That entire process lessens stress. Less stress promotes healing.

Self-love is so critical to our emotional and physical well-being, yet unless a person was raised with this inherent trait, few know how to achieve self-love on their own.

One of the times I noticed the probability that I had already developed a pretty healthy sense of self was when I was first stricken with rheumatoid arthritis and lived with the debilitation, deterioration and pain. I didn't like it one bit. So, I thought to myself, "Unless God means to kill me with this disease. He needs to deliver options to help me. I can't believe He really wants me to suffer like this." I continued, "I'm going to find these options because I don't deserve this. I deserve to be well." Somehow I knew it was all right to feel healthy, to be contented, and to have a good life. I could not have felt like that if I felt unworthy. This realization helped catapult me into not just one but several holistic healing journeys to deliver on that desire. In the process, I began to love myself to an even greater extent, which enhanced my life.

There is something wonderful that happens even if we realize we might not love ourselves enough. That realization gives us a place to start in learning this new concept. Yes, self-love can be learned. Even if you do not concentrate on it intently throughout your journey, it will come to you in the course of following the process outlined earlier in this book. As you begin to nurture yourself, your self-love and self-respect will grow. As you begin to make more of an investment in your health, focusing on your needs will become easier. In the process, the love you currently have for yourself will expand and as your choices improve, you will see stressors fall away and peace and contentment flood into your life.

You will notice yourself thinking more independently not merely recycling the opinions of others. You will begin to form independent opinions about your work, your relationships and the values that guide your life. You may revise the goals you had set for yourself. The more independent your thoughts – the more you will generate self-esteem. Having your own opinions and being willing to share them is an empowering exercise. You don't have to be right - you don't have to fight to convince others - you just have to acknowledge that you are entitled to opinions of your own. And, you have a right to act on those opinions as long as they don't hurt anyone else.

In the process of developing beliefs or philosophies that govern your health, you may find they are not popular with others but you will learn to trust your inner feelings and to respond to what is right for you. You will also become stronger - sometimes by not saying much to others about what you are doing, but quietly doing it anyway. There is a strength that comes with doing something and not just talking about it. If you are lucky, you will have family and friends who support you, but if you do it alone you will grow even stronger.

Your path to wellness is paved with exercises to build your sense of self-worth and self-love. That path will help you follow your inner voice, learn to trust yourself and develop a passion for a better life. The sense of pride you will feel from your achievements is something no one can take from you. Each exercise in self-nurturing will also contribute to enhancing your self-love.

To possess self-esteem is to truly be independent inside. Self-esteem is an intimate experience; it resides in the core of our being. It is what we think and feel about ourselves, not what someone else thinks or feels about us.[30] When we possess authentic self-esteem or self-love, we are content and at peace with who we are. We don't concern ourselves with what others think.

As you experience the process of finding your love of self and allow yourself to rediscover who you really are, it will be quite fulfilling. It may take the courage at first to change outdated

---

[30] Nathaniel Branden, *The Power of Self-Esteem* (Deerfield Beach: Health Communications, Inc., 2001), 37.

beliefs but in doing so you will develop the willingness to recognize, and then to fulfill your own needs. Yes, this healing journey will give you a wonderful new perception of yourself and it will have other extraordinary benefits, as well.

Stress Will Be Reduced, Too

Better choices mean less exposure to people or things that cause stress. You will have the confidence to say "no" politely and therefore you'll put up with less. You will change and so will the people around you. Those who are meant to remain in your life will begin to treat you differently, with more respect. Those who are not meant to stay will fall away. As you love yourself more others around you will respond accordingly.

Over the years, I have held a number of workshops on stress and one key point that I make is how it is possible to identify how much self-love a person has by identifying how they are treated by others around them. If you are constantly abused, dismissed, talked down to, ignored, ridiculed or yelled at - you need to work on your own self-esteem. You may say, "That's impossible in an environment that is this unhealthy." Yet, it is true that if you change you and in this case, I'm speaking about the attitude about yourself, the things around you will also change. As you develop a healthier self-esteem, your tolerance level will shift and you will quit putting up with behavior that causes you discomfort or stress. It becomes easier to walk away.

So, in the process of finding your authentic self through your holistic healing journey, you will find healthier relationships, more personal pride and a deeper respect for who you are. Less stress is not only more peaceful, it is healthier. So, in the process of embracing this journey and following the roadmap set forth in this book, you will not only be regaining your health you have a better chance of retaining it in the future.

Gifts Delivered From Your Alone Time

As I moved through my journey, I noticed much more alone time popping up around me. The time, initially came in the form of sleepless nights because of pain and having too little energy to leave home. It came because I was unable to do anything for a period of time and was forced to rest for days or weeks on end. In addition, it also came because I actually learned to carve out precious time for nurturing myself. That valuable time will also appear for you through the gift of time and other gifts will also begin to appear.

The gift of reflection. A break in the action, which might be the first time you've had to reflect on circumstances and tackle self improvement.

The gift of practice time. Precious time for trial and error, a part of the journey. Time to practice saying 'no', to practice self-discipline in lifestyle changes and to practice formulating new ways of valuing yourself - all at a much slower pace.

The gift of releasing control. This precious slow-down could be the first time you have had to deal with something out of your immediate control. This journey is a time when you have been taken out of the game, so to speak. You have been benched. You aren't the quarterback any longer; you aren't calling all the shots. This time you are second team in the game of life. You are forced to sit on the sidelines and to respond to what is given to you. Yes, you'll be forced to let go and go with the flow. All that remains is trust, faith and your body to guide you.

The gift of intuition. Hopefully, you'll learn to meditate and to quiet your mind, as you do so, you'll become more accustomed to living in the present moment. Only then can you easily hear the whispers and receive the signals your body is sending. All these steps are the precursor to being able to recognize many more intuitive gifts and realizing your human potential.

Thoughts to Consider

Self-love is the cornerstone of a healthy self-esteem.

A person with healthy self-esteem makes better choices in life.

A healthy sense of self includes the pride of being and the determination to care for your own needs.

You can learn to love yourself.

Healthy self-esteem helps eliminate stress.

To accept who and what you are you need not approve of everything about you. You can change and improve.

187

Narcissism is self-love and a perfect prescription for behavior during a
healing journey.

The more you love yourself the less need
you will have for illness.

Steps to Take

Do things to nurture yourself every day.

Keep thinking independently – it will strengthen your sense of self.

Take time to realistically asses who and
what you are.

Use your alone time to reflect, release control and develop your intuitive gifts.

Reflect on the experience that shaped your
life. Reframe those which are painful
or unpleasant.

Take time away from others to do things just
for you.

Give yourself love every day.

CHAPTER THIRTEEN

The Final Reward

*From Teetering On The Edge -
To Finding Total Balance*

F inally, with more time, improved health, more spiritual connectedness and enhanced self-esteem that creates less stress - balance will appear. Often awareness of the need for that balance comes in the form of an "ah ha". A close friend of mine had been plagued with a series of health issues during a six-year battle with her health. First it was chronic fatigue, then it was fibroid tumors in her uterus, weight gain became an issue and finally, high blood pressure surfaced. She knew these were sig-nals, she just wasn't sure of the message.

After making a serious commitment to make changes in her life and a weekend away to reflect on what was happening to her, she began to see the light at the end of the tunnel. First, she was open to answers and after some therapy with a friend, she awoke one morning with a revelation. She sat up in bed and announced to herself, "I have needed these illnesses to *make* me take time for myself. I spend my life taking care of others and only when I am ill - do I nurture *me*."

But, how do you find the time - or make the time? And then what do you do with the time, once you have it. What does balance look like in your life? As we ask ourselves these questions, many answers will surface over the coming months. The rest of this chapter should help you focus on that need for balance and build awareness to accelerate the process of finding those balance points in your life.

Balance And Common Sense

Any well-balanced lifestyle is comprised of a number of opposites to enhance our healing - such as giving and taking and rest and exercise. With these two as perfect examples, let's explore the options. In giving and taking, for example, there are people who take from themselves to give to others and may suffer in the process, these people must also learn to love themselves more and give more to themselves. They must learn to receive. For the people who might be considered "takers", self-centered individuals who always seem to come first in their lives, they must learn to give of themselves to others through their actions, time and love. The balance they gain, primarily through developing self-love, will enrich the quality of their lives and help them increase their capacity to give to others.

Rest and exercise one would think is pretty much a matter of common sense, however, for some it is not. There are people who honestly believe exercise will make them well and even with an aggressive cancer, they push themselves to exercise - believing a strong physical body will help them heal. Wrong. Wrong. Wrong.

Again, while we need to move around enough so blood circulates in our veins and our lymph system gets stimulated regularly when we are very ill, we also need our rest. I found for me in the beginning it was 90 percent rest and 10 percent movement. The ratio adjusts as your body is ready and as you are feeling up to it. Never should you push through pain to heal (unless it is orthopedic related physical therapy). Your body should respond positively to everything you do - which is why it is so easy to discern why so many drugs are so harmful overall because our bodies react so negatively to them. If your body wretches and vomits - it doesn't take a genius to figure out, it is rejecting the method being used. Healing work should happen in peace, contentment, and with ease to the body. Your body will dictate the amount of exercise and rest it needs – always. We all need the following:

> Enough sleep so your body feels rested when you awake. Regardless of how many hours that turns out to be each night.

> Healthy, nutritious food, which your body tolerates well, eaten in moderate quantities for fuel and rebuilding. We should savor each bite, enjoy the experience, and give thanks for what we ingest.

> Supplements that balance whatever is lacking in your normal food intake or is not well assimilated routinely within your particular body chemistry.

> Some form of movement like aerobic exercise, massage or walking to keep the blood circulating through our veins and our lymph system flowing.

> At least eight glasses of water, a day to hydrate your systems and keep your body functioning properly.

A peaceful environment in which to exist - free of stress -that is also calm and nurturing.

If we are free from disease and living a relatively routine life, we still need active exercise and as we age, to maintain balance. If we enjoy in a glass of wine or cocktail, on occasion, perhaps a cigar or a little caffeine, moderation is the key. Prescription drugs and chemicals in food are also easier to tolerate, in moderation as well. Again, balance is the operative word.

Any drug or chemical ingestion, more than moderate consumption should be neutralized with castor oil packs over the liver (an Edgar Cayce remedy), detoxing baths, steams or saunas, the milk thistle herb or other methods to provide relief for your liver and to eliminate any residual toxins from your system.

Another key factor is your time and how you spend it. It should also reflect balance:

Quiet time each day for reflection, meditation or prayer.

Time to live your joy. To do things that delight you and make you truly happy and make you smile spontaneously when you think of or experience them.

Time to give to others: to volunteer, to nurture those in need, and to contribute your talents to help others less fortunate or in distress.

Time to unleash your creative self. Finding ways of self expression in which you will feel self-fulfilled and energized. It can be cooking, writing, arts or crafts, gardening, singing or dancing, woodworking restoring antiques. We all have creative gifts that help us express who we are. We must find time to identify those and to begin to express them.

Time to give to and to receive from others.

Time for appreciating yourself and the achievements you've accomplished measured through your income, other success or recognition.

Your life should also be spiritually and emotionally balanced, as well. With increased time, you will find more room for a spiritual connection that makes you comfortable and secure. Balance emotionally requires living a life that is not filled with dramatic highs and lows but one that flows effortlessly and peacefully. You will fall more easily into that flow once stress is removed and you feel more of a sense of connectedness.

Our bodies are the best determination of how in balance we are and will let us know when we need relief from the following:

If we feel rushed and frantic, we are out of balance.

If we feel driven by our jobs so we are continually pressured and stressed, we are out of balance.

If we find ourselves rushing from airport to airport, gulping down fast food, drinking more alcohol than we should and pulling ourselves out of bed after only a few hours sleep, we are out of balance.

If we don't have time to connect with our family or friends, haven't found a passion or hobby or don't experience any time to play, we are also out of balance.

Through this journey, your feelings and your body will guide you toward a more balanced life. But you cannot be reminded enough about the need to carve out enough time for *yourself.*

Simplifying Helps Ensure Balance

In order to have enough time in your life to experience that which brings you joy - you need downshift your lifestyle and make the time. Elaine St. James, in her wonderful little book, *Simplify Your Life,* states it perfectly when she describes one of the catalysts which led her and her husband to make dramatic changes in their lives and for her to write this book. "We wanted to free ourselves from the commitments, the people, and the obligations that kept us from having time to do the things we really want to do. We made the decision early on to stop doing the things we'd always done because we felt we *should* do them. Not only has this increased the time we have for ourselves, but it has greatly reduced the stress that comes from doing things we don't want to do."[31]

I have selected only a small sample of the hints she shares in this literary treasure. These little nuggets will clearly free up time so you can take more time for you, for your passion, your reflection and your healing.

- Reduce the clutter. Clean-out, throw away.

- Change routines and become more efficient.

- Scale down - sell the damn boat.

- Turn off the TV.

- Stop the junk mail and cancel magazine subscriptions.

---

[31] Elaine St. James, *Simplify Your Life,* (New York: Hyperion Publishing, 1994), 5.

- Simplify gift-giving.

- If you don't like certain holidays, pass.

- Stop the busy work.

- Get up an hour earlier.

- Learn to meditate.

- Get rid of relationships that no longer work.

- Do one thing at a time.

- Just say no.

- If it's not easy, don't do it.

This summary doesn't do justice to the detail that awaits within her book, but in order to make time to find the balance you need in life, you need to begin making dramatic changes to simplify. If those changes mean spending one day a month in solitude or canceling your newspaper subscription, so be it. If it means that you quit trying to change people, which clearly takes endless hours of energy and fretting, you should do that as well. It might also mean finding time for friendships, too long ignored. Once you free up a little time, then you need to decide what to do with the new time you've found.

Let Go Of What's Not Working

One of the stumbling blocks that keep us from freeing up the time we need is the fear of letting go. All of us have relationships, projects or situations we deal with routinely that might not be "working". If that is the case, it is important to understand that "letting go of what's not working" has many benefits you can reap. First, the stuff that does not work takes more time - it wastes your time. Second, the stuff that does not work causes stress - and none of us need more of that. Finally, the stuff that does not work causes you to stay locked into routines that don't allow for growth, new experiences and different options. Letting go saves time, reduces stress and opens you to a world of new possibilities.

Another way to look at these situations is to spend more time doing the easy things and less time doing the difficult ones. Simply stated, quit swimming up stream. If things are not working, stop them. That includes projects that are a tremendous drain, enormous effort and never seem to get anywhere, and it includes friendships that create more problems than joys.

We have all heard the expression, when one door closes, another opens. So, to make room for the new, more energized, healthier you - you will have to let go of what is causing you additional stress. Let go of the unhealthy relationships, stresses on the job - or the job, itself, old ideas and beliefs and repressed emotions - more beneficial replacements will surface. Healing requires that we leave the parts in our life that no longer serve us. When you do, you will have the space for something better: positive people, better opportunities, and fun experiences.

By letting go, you release the emotions or experiences that have left you too exhausted to heal. You gain the time you need to begin to experience what you *love* to do. All these things will strengthen your immune system. You will free up time to balance your life with positive activities and people who bring you joy, and all of this will enhance your potential for wellness.

Discovering Your Passion

Living with passion strengthens your immune system and stimulates healing. In the process of following this journey, you should have more time to identify what truly brings you passion and to live it more fully. For many, it will come automatically. If it does do so for you, this section might help.

Some people connect living your passion with living your purpose. That might be true. That then begs the eternal questions: "Why am I here? What is it I am supposed to do?" "What is my real purpose in life?" It is impossible to address these questions without connecting spiritually - which also should be an automatic offshoot of following the holistic healing process. For many of us, the reason we are here is simply to express who we really are.

Each of us came with wonderful natural gifts. Those gifts or that gift is evident in everything throughout our life. We may be a great communicator (speaker or writer), a patient listener, a master organizer, highly creative in some form, loving of others, compassionate and kind, a teacher, or a number of other traits you could easily list. Those gifts we have been exhibiting since we were young. They are the traits other people always commented on. "There, Betty goes again - organizing everything." Or, "Joey, will you explain that to your friend?" "Let's put Sally in charge - she's a natural leader." If you think back, there is something you have always done that people have identified with you.

This trait should be natural and easy for you to do not one that is forced or that you have to practice. That gift can stand alone or be linked with a belief or a cause that has grown more important to you throughout your life. But, finding it doesn't have to mean finding a new job or reaching some potential for success that seems miles away. It can be as simple as reawakening your gifts, applying them to something you feel is important and then offering them in a way that benefits others.

Then, once you are able to use that gift to help others, you will feel more fulfilled and joyful. Part of that joy will come over time with the recognition that your life has value and meaning.

There is a direction each of us could take that would bring us true satisfaction, great happiness and a boundless feeling of self-worth. And, expressing that natural gift may change in the way it is expressed over the years or throughout a lifetime. Yet, it is always the same gift, the same talent. When you identify that - or even, realistically look at what you have already been doing - it is possible to find ways to share that talent with even more people. For example, a warm, compassionate loving woman who always gave those gifts to her young family and the neighbor children find that as these children have grown away, she is left with no obvious receivers for the gifts she offers. One of many answers: she could offer to volunteer at a local children's hospital nurturing ailing children.

Exercising your talent helps generate the kind of feeling that makes you excited to wake up each morning. The kind that fills you with daily gratitude for the joy you feel and the love you share with others. If you still aren't sure what your "gift" is - ask your Higher Self, a Higher Power or God. When you have done that you will receive the answer. Once you begin to realize and live your joy your life will dramatically change and your health will also improve.

Greg Anderson is an author who created wellness in his life after being diagnosed with a deadly lung cancer. In his book, *The 22 (Non-Negotiable) Laws of Wellness*, Greg tells of a man named Roger Burtonelli who was diagnosed with metastic lymphoma and, confined to his room, was receiving morphine intravenously to manage the pain. His continual improvement began once he realized his wisdom gained through life could be shared with his grandchildren through letters. He shared the lessons he had learned in his life on a range of subjects from persistence and the value of reading to handling failure. Even in the face of what seems a hopeless situation, our spirit can soar if we are allowed to create, express and help others through our gifts.[32]

We have all seen people literally "come alive" when they begin a project that brings them joy and makes them feel fulfilled. It might be knitting afghans for family members or for those less fortunate, it might be joining the church choir or it might be planting a garden. Whatever it is for you, I can promise you this: on the days you are able to express that passion, you will wake up with an excitement and eagerness to begin, you will lose track of time while submerged in your new activity and you will feel fulfillment at every stage.

Your passion need not be a full-time commitment, it can be an avocation. Regardless of how your gift is expressed, it can become part of the balance in your life that allows you to truly demonstrate who you are and make it possible for you to help or bring joy to others.

---

[32] Greg Anderson, *The 22 (Non-Negotiable)Laws of Wellness*, (New York: Harper Collins Publishers, 1995), 160-161.

Forgiveness Adds Balance, Too

Because we are all mere mortals, we have all experienced anger, resentment and guilt many times throughout our lives. Some of these emotions we have held on to and never learned to adequately release. Since these are the most common and destructive feelings we can experience - we all need to find ways to balance or neutralize these emotions.

Forgiveness is one of the best tools to offset past angers, resentments and, yes, even guilt. If we can learn to forgive others and forgive ourselves, we will be able to release many negative emotions fueling the illnesses we now experience.

A number of authors, who bring insight to the healing process, all make reference to forgiveness as a key element in establishing wellness. Gerald G. Jampolsky, M.D., devoted an entire book to this subject, *Forgiveness - The Greatest Healer of All*. This is an incredible book that is short and a quick read. Louise Hay, in *You Can Heal Your Life*, states that we must choose to release the past and forgive everyone, ourselves included. We may not know how to forgive, and we may not want to forgive; but the very fact we say we are willing to forgive begins the healing process.[33] An affirmation she recommends: "I forgive you for not being the way I wanted you to be. I forgive you and I set you free." This affirmation sets *us* free.[34]

---

[33] Louise Hay, *You Can Heal Your Life,* (Carlsbad:Hay House 1987), 13.

[34] Louise Hay, *You Can Heal Your Life,* (Carlsbad: Hay House 1987), 14.

Christiane Northrup, M.D., also believes that forgiveness frees us. It heals our bodies and our lives, but it is also the most difficult step we must take in our healing process.[35]

Forgiveness cannot begin if we kid ourselves about our past and the hurts or suffering we have endured. We must realistically acknowledge the pain in our lives, realize the source of that pain and then move forward to forgive the person whoever inflicted that pain.

Dr. Northrup continued, "I recently saw a woman with migraine headaches that were becoming increasingly severe. She also had chronic vaginitis, multiple allergies, and a host of other problems too numerous to mention. A perfectionist, she routinely took on too much at her job. When she spoke, she formed her words in a careful and controlled way - and her face twitched in an exaggerated way. On her intake form, she noted that her father, maternal grandfather, paternal grandfather, three brothers, and all her uncles were alcoholic and that her mother had expected her to be an adult almost since birth." I was never allowed to play. I had to keep the house neat," she wrote. She firmly believed that "none of these alcoholics had any effect on me during the time I was living at home." Her denial was very clearly in place, while her body was screaming to get her attention. Forgiveness of her parents would be ridiculous in her case. It would simply be used to build up another layer of intellectual armor. This woman first has to acknowledge that she was adversely affected by her parents'

---

[35] Christiane Northrup, M.D., *Women's Bodies Women's Wisdom,* (New York: Random House, Bantam Dell Publishing Group,1994), 532.

behavior. Forgiveness is completely premature when a woman doesn't even acknowledge that she *has* an emotional abscess, let alone that it needs to be drained.[36]

Dr. Northrup concluded by saying, "True forgiveness, on the other hand, changes us at a core level. It changes our bodies. It is an experience of grace. As I write about this concept, I'm moved to tears by the holiness of what forgiveness really is."[37]

If we can picture situations in our life that were painful to us, acknowledge hurt and see the person who inflicted that pain - then we can begin to forgive them. There are also a number of guided meditation exercises that you can buy on tape or can be coached by any life coach specializing in work through the Course in Miracles that will make great inroads fairly quickly for forgiveness. If this is an area where you want improvement - just ask for help and answers will come.

Releasing negatives so that more positives can flow into your life, finding time to hear the messages your Higher Self will send, appreciating a new and stronger spiritual connection, finding more love and appreciation for yourself and others and effortlessly flowing with the process that eventually leads to complete healing are extraordinary side-effects of a holistic healing journey. Now, perhaps, you can see why I have become such an advocate of this option to wellness.

---

[36] Christiane Northrup, M.D., *Women's Bodies Women's Wisdom,* (New York: Random House, Bantam Dell Publishing Group,1994), 534.
[37] Christiane Northrup, M.D., *Women's Bodies Women's Wisdom,* (New York: Random House, Bantam Dell Publishing Group,1994), 534.

I will be praying for each of you as you enter this magnificent arena and know that the blessings you will enjoy will be more than your heart could ever imagine. Enjoy your journey.

Thoughts to Consider

A balanced life will flow effortlessly.

Steps to Take

Post the list of "needs" on pages 277 and 228 - then monitor your lifestyle to make sure you are living a balanced life.

Balance any excess toxic exposure with gentle detoxing measures such as liver packs and soaking baths.

Make time for yourself.

Do things you love to do.

Simplify. Try a few of the hints on page 230 - 231. Post them as a reminder of things that might help.

Do the easy stuff. Quit swimming upstream.

Begin to unleash your creativity by using the special gifts you were given.

Let go of what is not working.

Do what brings you joy. Live your passion; if you can't do so in work, then do it as a hobby.

Practice forgiveness on yourself and others.

Nurture yourself - you deserve it.

Addendum

Alternative Or Complementary Options

E xploring the possibilities that exist outside the realm of conventional medicine is fascinating and offers myriad of options. Those options range from those currently being acknowledged by Western Medicine such as Acupuncture, Osteopathy, and Chiropractic to others which have survived for centuries such as Herbal Medicine, Ayurvedic Medicine and Essential Oil Therapy as well as many, many more.

Listed here are the most common alternative therapies with very short, brief descriptions of each. Read through the list. As you read slowly through the list, notice if you are being drawn back to one of two of the options, if your eyes dart to one title over another first, if you feel more comfortable reading about one of them or if you seem more interested in one over another. Those are probably the ones you should explore.[38]

---

[38] List Creation: Simon Mills, M.A. and Stephen J. Finando, Ph.D. *"New Choices in Natural Healing,"* (Emmaus: Rodale Press),11-158; "Alternatives in Healing", (New York: MacMillan), 47.
[38]Andrew Weil, M.D., *"Spontaneous Healing "*(New York: Alfred A. Knopf, Inc., 1995), 238-247; Various Internet resources.

243

Acupuncture – Developed in China at least 2,000 years ago this method uses needles strategically placed on the body to open the flow of vital energy or Qi (chee). This is believed to influence the balance of the body's natural health. Acupuncture is used for managing pain, relieve acute sinus infections, speed healing of joint injuries, as an anesthesia in surgery and dental work and many other specific conditions. Acupuncturists receive certification after training and may be licensed in some states.

Affirmations - Positive affirmations, written in first person and present tense, are a form of autosuggestion in which a statement of a desired outcome or condition is deliberately meditated on or repeated in order to implant that thought into the subconscious. Some recommend reciting them in a quiet and restful state with an expectation of the desired result and the accompanying feeling. It is believed that the most effective affirmations are those that are written and then spoken with some element of believability in their make-up.

Acupressure - Also developed in China, acupressure is the older, original technique, a Chinese home remedy to cure headaches, backaches, sinus pain, neck pain, eyestrain and menstrual cramps as well as pain of ulcers, help heal sports injuries, relieve insomnia and alleviate constipation and other digestive problems. Many cruise ships recommend wristbands using acupressure to stop sea-sickness. This form uses the finger and hand pressure instead of needles to stimulate the Qi (chee), this body's most basic healing energy.

Aromatherapy and Essential Oils - The use of essential oils as aromatherapy can be documented in ancient Egyptian hieroglyphics and Chinese and Eastern Indian manuscripts as well as the references in the Bible but it wasn't referred to as aromatherapy until the late 1920's. These oils are primarily applied topically or diffused. It is believed these oils increase cellular oxygen, promote immune function and open the subconscious mind, among many other things. Some use custom blends to alleviate fear, mitigate insomnia and reduce pain. Practitioners vary.

Ayurvedic Medicine - Originating with the sages of ancient India 5,000 years ago, this approach to physical health, mental clarity and spiritual fulfillment has been made popular in the United States by Deepak Chopra, M.D. This practice treats patients as identified by blending certain body types with emotional tendencies, intellectual styles and spiritual inclinations to create a detailed portrait of each type of individual. It is a methodology that treats holistically. There is no licensing procedure and no accrediting board for Ayurvedic practitioners. Finding a skilled Ayurvedic doctor takes some effort.

Chelation Therapy - A process by which chelating agents bind with heavy toxic metals such as cadmium, lead and mercury or others as well as minerals such as calcium and are excreted from the body. Chelation agents can be purchased over-the-counter and taken orally at home or can be administered intravenously under the supervision of a nurse, naturopath or physician. There are over 150 doctors in the U.S. that are certified by the American Board of Chelation Therapy.

Chiropractic - Started formally in 1895, this modality was originally invented by the ancient Greeks in 1250 B.C., who invented the techniques. This form of therapy specializes in treating muscular and skeletal disorders through manipulation of the spine. Spinal problems can interfere with the nerve supply and blood circulation to the rest of the body as well as cause physical pain. This is effective for acute musculoskeletal pain, tension headaches and recovery from trauma. Chiropractic therapy is provided by licensed chiropractors with the initials D.C. after their name.

Colon Therapy (Colonics) - A colonic is a form of hydrotherapy that gradually and gently cleanses the colon pockets and stimulates muscle tone. It is sometimes used to relieve symptoms when lower back pain is aggravated by a distended colon. This therapy is thought to help keep the colon free of bacteria since our diets today contain fewer stone-ground whole grains and high-fiber foods. Clinics associated with A.R.E. (Association for Research and Enlightenment - Edgar Cayce Foundation) provide such therapies as well as individual practitioners.

Feldenkrais Work - a system of bodywork, movements and floor exercises designed to retrain the central nervous system. This process is innovative, gentle and quite effective in rehabilitating victims of stroke, cerebral palsy, trauma and other serious disabilities. This very often is excellent an alternative to standard physical therapy.

Herbal Medicine - This practice treats disorders with medicines that are derived exclusively from plant materials. Practiced widely in Europe and the Far East, remedies are developed to suit each person's individual needs in order to help the body heal it-self. You might find Naturopaths, Ayurvedic practitioners and traditional Chinese medical practitioners as well as Holistic physicians utilizing this form of treatment.

Holistic Medicine - Practitioners who include M.D.'s, commonly referred to as M.D. (H), believe in treating the mind, body and spirit of the patient. Patients are encouraged toward personal responsibility and are actively involved in the healing process. This modality is very open to alternative methods. There is a national American Holistic Medical Association. There is no licensing requirement, but rather a common general philosophy about treatment and patient involvement.

Homeopathy - Over 200 years old, this system of diagnosis and treatment is based on the use of highly diluted remedies made from natural substances which trigger the body's own immune response mechanism. It is basically harmless because the medicines it employs are very diluted. Effective for a range of problems including allergies, skin and digestive ailments, rheumatoid arthritis, ear and upper respiratory infections gynecological problems and headaches. Practitioners may be M.D.'s, osteopaths, chiropractors, naturopaths, chiropractors or lay persons. There is licensing for these practitioners in very few states.

Hydrotherapy - First used by Hippocrates in the fourth century B.C., hydrotherapy has been part of the healing tradition of nearly every civilization from ancient Greece and Egypt to Rome, where virtually all medicine was practiced at the public baths. Today, modern water treatments include baths, cold water sprays, rubs, steam inhalation and hot and cold compresses. Internal uses range from enemas and colonics to drinking enough fresh, pure water every day to promote health. Spas provide some of these treatments; others may be prescribed by health practitioners.

Hypnotherapy - This modality takes advantage of the mind/body connection by placing the patient in a hypnotic state to heighten suggestibility that is geared toward affecting relief or a behavioral change. The best practitioners are inventive and willing to try new strategies to access spontaneous healing. Licensed hypnotherapists should be consulted.

Imagery and Visualization - This process has been considered a healing tool in virtually all the world's cultures including Western Indian tribes such as Navajos and the Ancient Egyptians and Greeks including Aristotle and Hippocrates. The power of "seeing yourself healthy" or specifically applying healing techniques in your mind's eye is well documented as effective. Imagery and visualization can be practiced in the privacy of your own home and with the aid of tapes or how-to manuals. No disease process is beyond the scope of guided imagery and visualization therapy for its potential is far reaching. Some people prefer to be led by a trained professional as in guided imagery.

Juice Therapy - Fresh juices can be potent weapons against disease and are considered natural tonics, which offer a safe, inexpensive way to stimulate digestion, bolster the immune system and encourage the elimination of toxins. This therapy is often used in conjunction with other natural techniques. You'll find

Ayurvedic practitioners and naturopathic physicians the most likely to recommend this remedy.

Massage - This is perhaps the most natural of natural remedies. Touching your body where it hurts seems to be a basic instinct. Swedish massage is the most common form, formally introduced in the nineteenth century although original forms of massage have been around for at least 5,000 years. The benefits of this treatment include reducing muscle tension, stimulating or soothing the nervous system, enhancing skin conditions, improving blood circulation, promoting better digestion and intestinal function, increasing mobility in joints, reducing swelling and inflammation and relieving chronic pain. Everyone should get routine massages. All states have licensed massage therapists.

Meditation and Relaxation - Relaxation and meditation techniques can boost immunity and lessen feelings of stress and anxiety. These techniques also reduce muscle tension, lower heart rate, blood pressure, metabolism and breathing and spark tranquil feelings. You can do them in your own home aided, initially by tapes or how-to manuals. Most forms of meditation use a picture, a word (mantra), an object (such as a candle flame) or a sensation (such as breathing) to focus the mind, The object is to clear your mind of useless clutter and to become more centered within.

Naturopathy - This form of treatment relies primarily on reforming the patient's diet and lifestyle. Based on Greek, Oriental and the old tradition of European health spas, patients find an emphasis on hydrotherapy, massage and nutritional and herbal treatments. Some chiropractors are also naturopaths. These physicians, who generally have a N.D. or N.M.D. after their name, may also use acupuncture, bodywork and homeopathy and are effective as advisors and helping people design healthy lifestyles. Some states license these practitioners and they are even able to issue medical prescriptions.

Nutritional Therapy - This modality goes as far back as Hippocrates who said in 400 B.C., "Let food be your medicine and medicine be your food." This practice does not rely solely on your daily food intake and may augment therapy with supplements since when food is processed or refined, it loses its nutritional punch. There are fewer vitamins and fiber, more fat and more sugar along with food additives which can cause many side-effects to people ingesting them. Some foods actually trigger a weakening of the immune system. A good nutritionist or naturopath can help you find a nutritional program that suits your particular body-type and metabolism and helps eliminate foods that may be damaging to your health.

Osteopathy - Physicians with the same educational background as M.D.'s but with additional training in manipulation practice this craft. It includes considering all parts of the body including treatment of the spine. These practitioners also work on all parts of the body. Cranial therapy is a specialized form of osteopathic medicine and is particularly beneficial for asthma, recurrent ear infections in children, sleep disorders and other conditions rooted in nervous system imbalances. Licensed in all states, Osteopaths can be differentiated by the D.O. which appears after their name.

Reflexology - although foot massages have been around since the beginning of time, this process for releasing stress and tension in the body by applying gentle pressure to certain areas of the feet, started in the early twentieth century. The founder was American doctor, William Fitzgerald, M.D. and later mapped by Eunice Ingham, an American massage therapist, who showed which spots on each food to touch to aid healing elsewhere on the body. Practitioners can be certified by the International Institute of Reflexology, the North American Association of Reflexation or Laura Norman and Associates, Reflexology Center.

Regression Therapy - Also called Past Life Therapy, occurs when a patient is hypnotized by a licensed hypnotherapist who also specializes in regressions. The patient is then asked to recall past lives. This type of therapy can quickly and effectively resolve many emotional problems, conflicts, fears and phobias usually in far fewer sessions than with conventional therapy.

Religious Healing - There is substantial research to support the beneficial effects of prayer in healing. Christian Science healing has been effective for years. Belief on the part of the patient is probably important, however, some research shows prayer to be effective even when sick people are unaware they are the objects of prayer. Prayer in healing knows no denomination.

Rolfing - This form of bodywork attempts to restructure the musculoskeletal system by working deep tissue in order to release patterns of tension. Rolfing can sometimes be painful and is used to release repressed emotions as well as to dissipate chronic or habitual muscle tension.

Shiatsu - A Japanese form of bodywork in which the practitioner uses firm finger pressure and applies it to specific points on the body. It is intended to increase the circulation of vital energy. This can also be painful if administered by traditional Japanese therapists. The Western form is more gentle.

Sound Therapy - About 2,500 years ago the Greek mathematician and philosopher, Pythagoras, developed "prescriptions" of music to help his students work, relax, sleep and wake up better. Some believe the sounds we make with our own voice have even more healing power than external sounds. "Toning" sounds, self-generated, can help one relax, ease stress and balance the body and mind. Today, sound is used to regulate heartbeat and ease pain. Some physicians use it to relax patients in surgery or for invasive diagnostic work.

Trager work - a gentle form of bodywork using rocking and bouncing motions to induce states of deep relaxation. This modality helps facilitate the nervous system's communication with muscles and is a particularly helpful rehabilitation therapy for people suffering from chronic neuromuscular problems, traumatic injuries and many other disabilities.

Traditional Chinese Medicine (TCM) - By observing various parts of the body, especially the tongue and pulse, practitioners provide treatment, which could include dietary change, massage, medicinal teas and other herbal preparations. TCM can be highly effective for an extremely wide range of conditions from auto-immune diseases including HIV and sexual deficiency to chronic degenerative conditions including Crohn's disease and chronic fatigue syndrome. Practitioners of Traditional Chinese Medicine (TCM) receive certification after training, and may be licensed in some states.

Vitamin and Mineral Therapy - The practice of treating various conditions of the body with vitamins and minerals. Because of the risk of creating imbalances, especially with some minerals and non-water soluble vitamins, it is best to get professional supervision from a naturopath, holistic physician or other health care professional trained in nutritional therapies.

Yoga - This practice, which is believed to have originated nearly 5,000 years ago, consists of breathing, stretching and meditation and can take only a few minutes each day but is valuable for releasing built-up tension and stress. It is intended to join or balance the mind, body and breath. You can take Yoga classes or practice in your own home with the aid of books or audio and video tapes.

To learn more about holistic healing,
about navigating the world of alternative medicine
and about helping yourself heal, visit:

www.sandycowen.com.